Should I Be Worried?

Dr Niamh Lynch is a consultant paediatrician living in Cork, Ireland.

Niamh graduated from University College Cork Medical School in 1998, where she won several awards, and completed her paediatric training in Temple Street Children's Hospital, The National Maternity Hospital Holles Street, the Rotunda Maternity Hospital, and Our Lady's Hospital for Sick Children, Crumlin.

In 2003, she volunteered with the United Nations and worked with UNICEF in Kathmandu, Nepal. In 2005 she commenced a fellowship in Paediatric Neurology in Vancouver, Canada.

Since 2012, Niamh has been working at Bon Secours Hospital, Cork as a consultant paediatrician with a special interest in paediatric neurology. She is also part of the Paediatric Neurology team at Cork University Hospital.

Her interest in clear, accessible health communication led her to social media in 2021. During the Covid-19 pandemic, when access to GPs and public-health nurses was affected by lockdowns and restrictions, she began sharing fact-based information about child health on Instagram (@dr_niamh_lynch) and TikTok (@tiktokkiddydoc). Her social-media community has now grown to over 300,000 followers and she is a regular contributor to Irish media.

Niamh is married with two daughters and a house full of pets. Music is a big part of her downtime: she sings in a choir and is learning to play the ukulele (badly!).

Dr Niamh Lynch

Should I Be Worried?

A no-panic guide to your child's health

HACHETTE
BOOKS
IRELAND

Copyright © 2026 Niamh Lynch

The right of Niamh Lynch to be identified as the Author of the Work has been asserted by her in accordance with the Copyright, Designs and Patents Act 1988.

First published in Ireland in 2026 by
HACHETTE BOOKS IRELAND

2

All rights reserved. No part of this publication may be reproduced, stored in a retrieval system, or transmitted, in any form or by any means without the prior written permission of the publisher, nor be otherwise circulated in any form of binding or cover other than that in which it is published and without a similar condition being imposed on the subsequent purchaser.

Cataloguing in Publication Data is available from the British Library

ISBN 9781399746717

Typeset in Source Sans Pro by
Palimpsest Book Production Ltd, Falkirk, Stirlingshire

Printed and bound in Great Britain by
Clays Ltd, Elcograf S.p.A.

Hachette Books Ireland policy is to use papers that are natural, renewable and recyclable products and made from wood grown in sustainable forests. The logging and manufacturing processes are expected to conform to the environmental regulations of the country of origin.

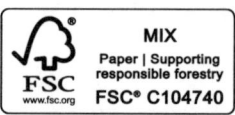

Hachette Books Ireland
8 Castlecourt Centre
Castleknock
Dublin 15, Ireland
(info@hbgi.ie)

Authorised representative in the EEA

A division of Hachette UK Ltd
Carmelite House, 50 Victoria Embankment, London EC4Y 0DZ

www.hachettebooksireland.ie

This book is dedicated to my husband and my two daughters.

The information in this book is not intended to replace or conflict with the advice given to you by your GP or other health professional. All matters regarding your or your child's health should be discussed with your GP or other health professional and you should always seek medical advice if you have any health concerns. The author and publisher accept no responsibility from the use of the material in this book by any person.

The information contained in this book is, to the best of the author's knowledge, accurate at the time of publication. Readers should confirm all such information at the point of using it to ensure it is still up to date.

Contents

Introduction — 1

Part I
What to Expect: Ages Zero to Five

1: The First Week — 13
2: 2 to 6 Weeks — 40
3: 7 to 12 Weeks — 66
4: 4 to 6 Months — 82
5: 6 to 12 Months — 104
6: 1 to 2 Years — 130
7: 2 to 5 Years — 154

Part II
Health Concerns in the Early Years

8: Tummy Troubles — 197
9: Developmental Differences — 209
10: Is This Something Serious? — 221
11: Fits, Faints, and Funny Turns — 247
12: Hospital Visits and Doctors' Appointments — 267

13: Teething and Teeth	275
14: Skin and Rashes	283
15: A to Z	294
Acknowledgements	381
Image credits	382
Resources	383
Index	385

Introduction

Hello, and welcome to my book! My name is Dr Niamh Lynch and I am a paediatrician working in Cork. This book is all about child health – what is normal, what is concerning, and what you can expect from the moment your baby takes their first breath.

How this book came about is a tale of how I finally managed to combine the language of medicine and motherhood into a straightforward guide to your child's health.

The story began in my first anatomy class. I sat with 80 other fresh-faced medical students as our professor cast his cool gaze across the room.

'You will learn as many new words in this semester as a student learning Russian for a year.' There was a collective raising of eyebrows. 'Those of you who studied Latin in school are at a slight advantage,' he continued, and the Latin scholars smirked. 'Alas,' he sighed, looking directly at one of the smirkers, 'Ancient Greek is no longer on the curriculum, so you will all struggle equally with many of the anatomical terms.' All grins drained away. 'Now, let's begin.'

Over the coming years, we learned the names and precise location and function of every part of the human body, from synapse to synovium, vena cava to villi. Then, we learned about how disease and dysfunction affect the body's organs and systems. By the time I graduated, a sentence such as, 'The patient is pyrexial, tachycardic and hypotensive with suspected

2 | SHOULD I BE WORRIED?

bacteraemia and hypovolemia' made total sense to me and my classmates.

We had gone into medical school speaking plain, simple English; we graduated speaking an entirely different language. The weird thing is, not one lesson focused on how to translate this medical jargon back into plain English. At no point were we specifically taught how to communicate with the patient (or parent) in front of us. (This was a long time ago and, thankfully, things have improved in recent years.)

With my head full of jargon and my heart in my mouth, I was launched on to the hospital wards as an intern. I was young and completely green. Far from the austere professors in medical school, I acquired a new set of teachers: my nursing colleagues, the clerical staff, the domestic staff, and the patients and their families.

After my year of internship, I was just about mastering the art of communicating in a clear and compassionate way with adult patients. Then I got my place on a paediatric training scheme – and it was time to learn a new language.

In July 1999, I made my way down the side alley to the paediatric emergency department of Temple Street Children's Hospital in Dublin, and nervously introduced myself to the receptionist, who smiled warmly and directed me to a room full of equally nervous-looking young doctors. We nodded awkwardly at each other and stood in silence, which was interrupted by the sounds of newborns crying and children laughing. Then, the door burst open and in came my newest teacher. This was a doctor unlike any I had met before. His face was creased from smiling and his jokes were hilarious. Then, he got serious. 'You only have two things to learn here. The first is that by the end of month one, you need to know the difference between "sick" and "well". The second is you are never the person with the most important thing to say. The parents are the ones saying the important stuff. Oh, and one more thing ... you need to know what "lobbin' and lyin'" means. Welcome to Dublin!' And out he skipped. Dr Peter Keenan – Ireland's very first consultant in paediatric emergency medicine, and the first of many inspiring teachers I was to meet on my journey through paediatrics.

I was left wondering, what did he mean by 'sick' or 'well'? Surely all children coming to the emergency department were sick in some way or another. And what on earth was 'lobbin'' and lyin''? I was soon to learn the answer to those questions in the form of a little three-year-old boy.

'What seems to be the problem?'

'I'm not sure, Doc. He's been lobbin' and lyin' for the last three days. He's vomiting since this morning. He's just not right.'

The little boy peered at me from big, sunken eyes.

'Any diarrhoea?'

'No.'

'Is he peeing?'

'Yeah, non-stop.'

'Is he eating and drinking?'

'He won't eat for me. But he's fierce thirsty.'

Having dealt with about 10 cases of gastroenteritis that week, I had already drawn my conclusion. This was a simple case of a tummy bug. We would give him oral rehydration fluids, and he would be as right as rain in a few hours. I explained my plan to his mother, who looked dubious. 'I think he'll just vomit up that drink, Doc.'

'Let's give it a try and, if it doesn't work, we'll come up with a new plan.'

We placed the little boy, quiet and drowsy, onto the bed. I thought I had a few hours to treat him and observe his response. What I didn't realise was that we were actually in a situation where time was of the essence. I wasn't working alone and, to this day, I thank my lucky stars that the senior nurse in the treatment room could see something was seriously amiss. She saw true sickness, where I saw a tummy bug.

'Niamh,' she said quietly, sitting next to me as I wrote up my treatment plan, 'do you think we should check a urine sample before I start his fluids?'

4 | SHOULD I BE WORRIED?

'Of course,' I said nonchalantly, and then I froze. Tired, thirsty, sore tummy, huge volumes of urine ... I knew then that there was going to be glucose in that urine. This child had undiagnosed diabetes and was probably in diabetic ketoacidosis. This was a life-threatening scenario, and we had to act quickly. I swallowed hard.

'You're thinking diabetes, aren't you?' I croaked. 'Oh my God, how did I miss it? I'll get IV access and send off the bloods. Can you call the rest of the team and let Dr Keenan know?'

With a hammering heart, I explained to his mum that the plan had changed and that we needed to put in some IV cannulas and do some more tests. The toddler barely moved as I pushed large needles into his veins. This child was sick, and I had nearly missed it. As we all worked quickly to stabilise this little boy, Dr Keenan appeared by my side. 'Diabetic ketoacidosis,' he said, one eyebrow cocked. 'Nice pick-up, Dr Lynch. He's going to be fine.'

'It wasn't me who picked it up,' I said, somewhat shamefaced at my near miss, 'it was Margaret, the nurse.'

He laughed.

'Do you really think it's a coincidence that we put the most junior doctors with the most senior nurses? The important thing is you listened. And today you learned the difference between "sick" and "well".'

I still didn't really know what 'lobbin' and lyin'' meant and, to this day, I don't know how you would translate it exactly. It's not something I ever heard in Cork hospitals. But I had learned that when a Dublin parent used this phrase, they were worried about their child, and they were telling me something very important.

As my training in paediatrics went on, I got better at communicating with parents. I learned from another great teacher, Professor Anthony Ryan, that sometimes what is not said carries far more weight than what is, because some worries are just too enormous for parents to say out loud. He taught me to ask parents, 'What are you most worried about?', and it was amazing to me how much they would share when asked so directly. I learned that listening is communicating, and how much parents value that feeling of being listened to.

Three years into my paediatric training, just when I had got somewhat proficient in listening to and speaking with families, I undertook a long-standing promise to my granny. Before she died, she asked me to put my medical skills to use in less wealthy countries, where poverty was a barrier to healthcare. So, I signed up as a United Nations volunteer and headed to Kathmandu, Nepal, to work with UNICEF.

This was how I found myself in the foothills of the Himalayas without a word of Nepali, working with village health workers. These incredible women were volunteering for their community, taking on the responsibility of visiting sick children, administering medications, and providing crucial advice on vaccines and nutrition. Although we did not share a language, we shared a purpose – and we shared many, many laughs. These women showed me what it was like to have a true passion for the health of your own community. In remote mountainous areas, where there were no health facilities or hospitals, these women delivered life-saving care with nothing in their medical kits except a thermometer and a stopwatch to count a child's heart rate and breathing rate.

Coming back to Ireland was a bit of a culture shock. We were in the peak of the Celtic Tiger and conspicuous consumption was the order of the day. It was such a contrast with my simple life in Nepal. However, there was no time to dwell on this, as I was straight in to acquiring a new set of skills in a new and unfamiliar hospital. This time, I was in the sprawling Our Lady's Hospital for Sick Children in Crumlin – or, as we all knew it, 'Crumlin'. I immediately noticed one big difference on the south side of Dublin city compared with Temple Street Hospital in the north inner city. In just a few short miles across the River Liffey, the language of concern changed. No one said 'lobbin' and lyin''; here, it was the phrase 'thrown down' that would set alarm bells ringing when uttered by a parent.

6 | SHOULD I BE WORRIED?

At this time, I was also learning my craft in paediatric neurology, my chosen speciality. I learned new terms and diagnoses. I watched as my next great teacher, Professor Joe McMenamin, gently guided parents through life-changing times, speaking softly and kindly in his Donegal accent. Like other wonderful paediatricians I had met, Professor McMenamin listened more than he spoke. Because neurology is a speciality where the diagnosis is often elusive, he would take away a tiny detail of what a parent had told him and dispatch me like a detective to the library with this little nugget of information to scour journals and textbooks looking for more clues. This was in the time before rapid internet search engines and advanced genetic testing but, with those seemingly small pieces of information, we were able to find a diagnosis. Much has changed since then, but parents are still the ones in the room with the most important things to say.

In 2005, I was accepted on to a two-year neurology fellowship programme in Vancouver, Canada, and it was time to move again. By now, I had a much-loved dog and a much-loved fiancé, and the three of us headed off on our adventure to the west coast of Canada. Although they speak English in Canada (and French, of course), the vocabulary is different. In work, I took the 'elevator' and not the 'lift'. But I was never offered a 'lift' home, that was a 'ride'. When writing my notes in the hospital charts, I would leave 'orders' not 'requests'. Although the words they used were different, the parents, just like parents anywhere in the world, wanted to talk and wanted to be heard.

During my time in Canada, I uttered two very important two-word phrases of my own. In 2006 I said 'I do' and in 2007 I said 'I'm pregnant'. It was time for me to learn the language of parenthood.

You can spend eight years training as a paediatrician and still feel utterly incompetent when your own baby is handed to you. That was the case for me, anyway. I held so many facts about babies in my brain, but I had never before felt what becoming a mother did to your mind and body. And I didn't have the language for these first-time feelings. I didn't have words for the profound contentment in my new role as mother, or the constant low-grade anxiety about my baby's health and well-being. I didn't have words for the dazzling joy that came with her first smile, or the crushing exhaustion that came with colic and sleepless nights. I didn't have words, but I was gaining understanding. I was starting to understand that every parent I had ever encountered in my time as a young paediatrician had these feelings too. I was being schooled all over again, and I knew that when I went back to work after maternity leave, I was going to be a very different kind of doctor.

When I did return to work, I was no longer the new kid on the block. It was time for me to step up my responsibilities and become a consultant. My words suddenly felt heavier, as if they carried more weight. While I could talk to my consultant colleagues and ask for advice, when it came down to it, the conversations I had with parents about their child's diagnosis and prognosis were going to have added significance now that I was in a senior role.

I felt a great responsibility towards the children in my care, and a huge obligation to communicate well with parents at the most stressful time in their lives. I remembered the lessons I'd learned along the way: that I was never the person with the most important things to say, that listening is communicating, and that the smallest details shared by parents can be a huge help in figuring out a diagnosis. Most of the time, I think I did a good job. Sometimes, I know I didn't. I am still learning from colleagues, parents and children – both other people's children and my own!

One of the more recent things that I have learned from younger colleagues, and, indeed, from my teenaged children, is that the world has a whole new way of communicating now. If you had asked me in 2020 what the word 'content' meant, I would have said that a newborn snoozing in his mother's arms with a full belly and a freshly changed nappy was content. You know, happy, comfortable. Content.

Then, during the pandemic, when parents were struggling to get their children seen by a doctor or their baby's developmental checks done by a public-health nurse, I decided to create an Instagram account with information about child health for parents and caregivers. My own godson had just been born, and his parents shared with me the stresses they were feeling with a tiny baby in the house. I thought an Instagram page with reliable facts on child health might be some help to parents who felt isolated at that time. It was a spur-of-the-moment thing, done in the depths of a winter lockdown, and I was sure it would be a flash in the pan – but suddenly I had 1,000 followers, then 10,000. And now, more than 100,000.

The reason for this is still something of a mystery to me, but the one message (or 'DM', in social-media parlance) that I kept getting was, 'I love your content'. And I learned that 'content' is a word for the stuff you have on your Instagram (or TikTok or any other social media) page. And the stuff I have on my Instagram page just happens to be information. Facts. Reassurance. The words of healthcare spoken in the language of parents. Because back in 2021, more than anything else, I was a parent worried about my kids, just the same as everyone else.

Part of my job as a paediatric neurologist is spotting patterns – patterns in sleep, patterns in behaviour, patterns in scans. This helps me to help children by coming to a diagnosis. And now that I am active on social media and interacting with potentially tens of thousands of people whenever I put up a post, I am seeing different kinds of patterns. I am seeing a pattern of the same questions and worries from parents over and over again.

'Is this behaviour normal?'

'How will I know if my baby is really sick?'

'Do I need to take my toddler to the hospital?'

These are the worries that parents turn over and over in their brains. These are the worries that turned over and over in my brain almost 18 years ago when I held my first baby. And if there is one thing I have learned about worry, it is that articulating it – saying it out loud – turns it into a question.

Which led me here. I had to write this book. I had to write it because it felt like on social media, a parent was only ever three clicks away from a post that was utterly panic-inducing. This is because most social media exists only with engagement in mind, and posts that provoke fear or outrage drive engagement. Social media can be wonderful, but it is also a worry factory. I was seeing a pattern of parents getting more and more concerned about their kids, as the algorithm fed them dubious content. I had to use my words, my knowledge, and my experience – both as a paediatrician and as a parent – to write something that would bring reassurance and empowerment, not fear.

This is a book full of questions, not worries. It is a book full of advice, not alarm. It is a book written in your language and in my language. It is a 'no panic' guide to your child's health, and I hope you find it helpful.

PART I
What to Expect: Ages Zero to Five

In this first section of the book, we will lay the foundation for understanding your child's health and development in their vital first five years. As a consultant paediatrician with over 25 years of clinical experience (and just as importantly, as a mother), I know first hand how challenging it can be to interpret what's 'normal' and what might require medical attention.

This section is designed to help you feel more confident as a parent by guiding you through the key areas of your child's early life: crying, sleeping, feeding, growth, and development. These are the building blocks of early childhood health, and they're also the most common areas where parents have questions, concerns, or moments of self-doubt.

We'll begin by exploring what's typical at various ages and stages – how much crying is normal, how sleep patterns evolve, how feeding can change over time, what to expect from physical growth, and how developmental milestones unfold. You'll find reassurance in understanding the broad range of behaviours and timelines that exist in early childhood.

But knowing when things aren't going as expected is just as important. That's why this book also includes clearly outlined red flags – the signs and symptoms that suggest your child may need medical review, either by a GP, public-health nurse, or in hospital. Whether it's persistent feeding difficulties, unusual patterns of crying, developmental delays, or anything else that doesn't sit right with you, I want you to feel empowered to seek help.

I've written this with both my professional and personal hats on. I have information that I want to share with you, but I also know what it's like to stand in your shoes, searching for answers in the middle of the night. I want to help you feel informed, supported, and less alone on this marvellous journey called parenthood.

CHAPTER 1
The First Week

Your baby has arrived (or perhaps even babies!) and now, here you are, holding your newborn, and wondering ... what next? How am I going to care for this tiny human? How do I know if I am doing it right? Or doing it wrong?

The very first thing you need to know is that, if you're feeling lost or overwhelmed, don't worry – you are not alone! Most, if not all, parents of a new baby feel the same way. So let me guide you through the first week of your baby's life. You're setting out on a fantastic journey, and this will be your road map.

THE FIRST 24 HOURS

This first day can be intense. If you have birthed your baby yourself, then you have your own physical recovery to think of as well. Accept all the help offered by nurses, midwives, friends, and relatives. Rest, drink plenty of water, eat well, and remember to think of yourself in the midst of all the baby excitement.

But look at that little baby (or babies!). Aren't they just amazing? Hang on ... that noise they made. Was that normal? And, oh my goodness, *what* is in that nappy?

Let's get into it!

Breathing

The thing we all wait for as your baby emerges into the world is that first breath. All sorts of magic happen with this first breath. The lungs fill with air, the circulation in the heart changes, your baby starts to change colour, and their lips become rosy red. The first breath is usually announced with a cry and, with that cry, everyone else in the room breathes a sigh of relief.

When your baby has taken his or her first breath, they will usually be handed to their parents. If breastfeeding is planned, the midwife may suggest that your baby is placed on the mother's breast. Your baby might start to feed, they might simply stare at you intently, or they might take a quick look at you and decide to have a nap. All this time, the midwife is keeping an eye on your baby's colour and their breathing pattern, making sure that their lips look nice and pink, and that their breathing is not laboured in any way.

When you leave the labour ward – or, if you had a home birth, when the midwife leaves – you will probably start to observe your baby closely. With breathing, you want to see an easy pattern. It should look effortless and it should be silent. If you notice your baby grunting or groaning as they breathe, ask for them to be reviewed by a nurse or doctor.

Depending on your baby's skin colour, their hands or feet may look quite blue or purple for the first 24–48 hours. This is normal. However, if you see a blue or purple colour on your newborn's lips, ask that they be reviewed.

What if ...

What if the first breath, the first cry, doesn't come? About 10% of babies will need some help to begin breathing on their own. This happened to me with my first baby. After a long labour and tough delivery, she was, as the obstetrician described, 'stunned'.

Here's what happens if the first breath does not come, regardless of whether you have a hospital or home birth. Your baby will be taken by the midwife and dried quite vigorously. This stimulates the baby and, in the vast majority of cases, it's enough to get things going. If not, your baby might be given some oxygen or some puffs of air via special equipment. Most of the time, your baby then announces their arrival with a hearty cry!

What if baby still has difficulty breathing? If your baby is born in hospital, a team of doctors and nurses will arrive to help, and your baby will most likely need to go to neonatal intensive care for medical assistance and tests. If your baby is born at home, your midwife will be highly trained to deal with the situation, but will most likely call an ambulance and will have you and your baby transferred to hospital where you can both be taken care of.

Feeding

Babies will either be fed breast milk or formula (breast milk substitute). Breastfeeding has many benefits for both baby and mother, so, if baby can be breastfed for even a short period of time, give it a try. Breastfeeding needs support, so do avail of a lactation consultant if you have access to one in the maternity unit where your baby is born or in the community if you had a home birth.

Regardless of how baby is fed, we like to see two things in the newborn period: a good suck and a good swallow. Your baby's mouth should form a seal around the nipple (or bottle teat), with no milk escaping from their mouth. Their swallow should be easy, without coughing, spluttering, or gagging (they will have been practising their swallow in the womb since about week 14 of pregnancy!).

Some babies will want to feed every two hours, while others are content to wait for three to four hours. Your baby might bring up small amounts of milk after a feed. This is called 'posseting' and is to be expected. However, vomiting large amounts is not normal, neither is a green colour in the vomit – both of these situations need medical attention.

What if ...

What if my baby won't feed? If you are breastfeeding, you will get help and guidance from the midwives and, ideally, a lactation consultant. If your baby is having trouble with sucking or swallowing, regardless of how they are fed, they will be seen by a doctor and might need to go to the neonatal unit for some tests. Some babies, especially those who are small or whose mothers have diabetes, can have low blood sugar levels over the first few hours or days. Sometimes, the medical team will check sugar levels to look for this. If your baby is jittery (arms and legs shaky or shivery) between feeds, this could be a sign that their glucose levels should be checked.

Poop

You will never forget your baby's first poop! It is a sticky substance that can be black, brown, or dark green. This is meconium, a build-up of all the cells, mucus, and amniotic fluid that your baby has been swallowing since week 14 of pregnancy. Meconium should be passed in the first 48 hours. If your baby has not pooped in this timeframe, they will need a medical review during which they will be checked to make sure there is no blockage preventing them from opening their bowels.

When the meconium has passed, which might be over several nappies, the poop can take on a variety of colours and consistencies. Breastfed babies usually have yellowish, watery poops, whereas formula-fed babies tend to have more pasty, brown poops.

Pee

The first pee after birth is not as dramatic as the first poop! Your baby is a dab hand at peeing by the time they are born. The kidneys start to work at about week 11 of pregnancy, at which point your baby starts to pee. By week 20, most of the amniotic fluid (the fluid that surrounds your baby in the womb during pregnancy) has been through those kidneys. In the first 24 hours, your baby will probably have one or two wet nappies. The urine colour is usually light to dark yellow. If no urine has been passed in those 24 hours, baby will need a medical assessment where a doctor might check their fluid intake, and their kidneys and bladder.

Sleep

It is exhausting being born! Your baby will probably spend 13–19 hours of their first 24 hours asleep. After their first feed, they will usually settle into a sleep that can last a few hours. After this, they may develop a pattern of short sleeps (30–60 minutes), followed by waking for feeds. Their little tummies are small, and they will need to feed every 3–4 hours at least. Your baby also learned how to sleep in the womb, so they should be able to settle to sleep easily in the first 24 hours. If, in the first 24 hours, you cannot get your baby to sleep, or they seem very cranky or irritable, they should be medically reviewed.

Crying

Crying is very normal in newborns. In fact, it is their main means of communication: 'Waah! I'm hungry', 'Waah! I'm tired', 'Waah! Change my nappy', 'Waah! I need a cuddle'. At first all the cries might sound the same to you but, as time goes by, you will probably begin to understand what your baby is trying to tell you.

In the first 24 hours, a little bit of crying is to be expected but, remember, your baby will probably spend most of their first day asleep. Crying in the first 24 hours becomes a concern if it is continuous, high pitched, or if the baby is very irritable and won't settle. In this case, your baby will need to be medically reviewed.

Skin

Your baby's skin may appear quite blotchy in the first 24 hours. If you are in hospital, the nurses will be monitoring closely for signs of jaundice, but this isn't something to be concerned about until later in week one.

The umbilical cord

When the umbilical cord is clamped and cut, a few centimetres of cord remain attached to your baby's tummy, along with the plastic clamp. This is known as the umbilical stump. It starts to dry up very quickly and falls off by itself between days 5 and 15. While it is attached, keep it clean, and make sure to wash your hands before and after touching it. Fold the front of the nappy down so that it doesn't cover the stump. Do not pull at the stump – it will fall off by itself.

Routine health checks

Your baby's weight, height, and head size (circumference) will be recorded at birth. The midwife or doctor will check your baby's heart and lungs (pulse and oxygen levels), their eyes (very rarely babies can be born with cataracts), their mouth (for any evidence of a cleft palate), their hips (to screen for hip dysplasia), and their genitalia (to ensure they appear normal). They will also check to ensure that your baby is able to move both arms and both legs without difficulty. Sometimes a baby can sustain damage to the nerves that supply the arms during delivery and have weakness in the affected arm. This is known as Erbs palsy and will require specialised follow-up with paediatricians and physiotherapists. Within the first 24–48 hours, your baby will also have the newborn hearing screen. This is a straightforward test that involves putting a small earpiece on your baby's ear to check that they can hear okay. It's usually done when they are settled or asleep, and it can be repeated if needed.

> ### VITAMIN K
>
> Vitamin K is offered for all newborns at birth, with parental consent. This is usually given by injection into the thigh muscle. Vitamin K is vital for helping blood to clot, and babies have very low levels of it when they are born. Giving a dose shortly after birth prevents a very serious condition known as vitamin K deficiency bleeding (VKDB). This can lead to brain bleeds or even death. The risk of VKDB is 1 in 100 without vitamin K being administered; that risk falls to less than 1 in 10,000 when a baby has received a vitamin K injection.

CONGRATULATIONS!

You have just spent the first 24 hours with your newborn. Let's dive into week one and see what adventures await.

WEEK ONE

You might be reading this before your baby arrives or perhaps your baby has already arrived and you want to check something you are just not sure about! Either way, let's have a look at what is normal and *not* normal with your baby's feeding, poop, pee, sleep, crying, and skin in the first week of their lives.

Plus, a couple of surprising (some may even say weird) things, such as witch's milk and baby periods!

Feeding

In the first week, you and your baby will establish feeding. If you are breastfeeding, then there's a lot going on for you as well, with milk coming in (where your milk supply transitions from the initial colostrum to mature milk) and your boobs literally changing overnight. In general, milk will have come in by day five. This can seem very sudden, but your breasts have been producing a mix of colostrum (protein- and antibody-rich milk, sometimes called 'liquid gold' because it can be yellow in colour) and smaller amounts of breast milk before the supply suddenly increases.

What you are looking for with feeding in the first week, regardless of whether it is via breast or bottle, is that your baby is waking for feeds, is interested in feeding, and is latching on well.

It is hard to know how much volume your baby is getting if you are breastfeeding, but you should be able to hear them swallowing, they should be satisfied and seem full after a feed, and they should be having regular wet nappies (between five and six per day).

If you are bottle feeding, remember that your baby's stomach is very small, and they will feed little and often. In general, they will take 45 to 90 millilitres per bottle, and feed every 3–4 hours.

If you are breastfeeding and it is painful when your baby latches on, or if your baby cannot latch on well, then they will need to be assessed for tongue-tie.

TONGUE-TIE

The medical term for tongue-tie is ankyloglossia. Tongue-tie happens when the small band of tissue under a baby's tongue (the frenulum) is too short, tight, or placed in a way that limits tongue movement. This, in turn, may affect feeding.

In recent years, frenotomy, or 'tongue-tie release', has become an increasingly common procedure to perform on babies. This involves cutting the frenulum with a scissors, scalpel or laser.

As this is a surgical procedure, it is important that it is only performed when clinically indicated, and by appropriately qualified practitioners. Recently the Royal College of Physicians of Ireland and the HSE produced guidelines to help clinicians and lactation consultants decide when a frenotomy should be performed.

These guidelines recommend a multidisciplinary approach. Communication between paediatricians, lactation consultants, general practitioners, and public-health nurses is essential. International Board Certified Lactation Consultants (IBCLC) should perform a complete feeding assessment before a frenotomy is performed.

Why tongue-tie matters

Breastfed babies use their tongue to latch and draw milk. If it can't move well, feeding can be uncomfortable for both baby and mum. Signs can include painful nipples for the mother, long or ineffective feeds, slow weight gain, or frustration for baby.

Most babies with tongue-tie don't have serious issues, but for some, it can make breastfeeding harder. Not all babies with a visibly short or thick frenulum will need a frenotomy. It is only indicated if it is causing issues with feeding.

How tongue-tie is checked

Specialists (usually a lactation consultant) look at appearance (where the tongue attaches) and function (how it moves). They also watch your baby feed: is milk transferring well, is the person breastfeeding comfortable, is baby growing as expected? Special checklists or scoring tools are sometimes used to guide decisions.

When treatment is helpful

If tongue-tie is clearly linked to nipple pain in the mum and/or feeding problems in the baby, and support with positioning or latch hasn't solved things. Feeding usually improves right away, especially with follow-up help from a lactation consultant.

When treatment is NOT needed

If baby is feeding well, gaining weight, and mum is comfortable, no procedure is necessary, even if a frenulum looks tight. Doctors do not recommend 'just in case' procedures for ties that aren't causing trouble. There is not sufficient evidence that tongue-tie causes problems with speech or with teeth in later childhood.

Frenotomy is not usually recommended for babies who are bottle fed only. This is because the tongue and mouth movements a baby uses to take milk from a bottle are different to when feeding from the breast.

Regardless of how your baby is fed, if they are having trouble sucking or swallowing, are coughing, choking, or gagging when feeding, or getting out of breath, they will need to be seen by your public-health nurse or GP.

Winding a baby gently by rubbing or softly patting their back will help them to burp. They will often bring up a small amount of milk when they do. This is called posseting, and it is normal. However, if they are vomiting larger amounts after feeds, speak to your public-health nurse or GP.

Projectile vomiting is very different to regular vomiting and is a worrying symptom. With projectile vomiting, the vomit shoots out of the mouth and can land quite a distance from the baby. This can be a sign of a blockage in the stomach known as pyloric stenosis and it requires urgent medical review and treatment.

Vitamin D

Vitamin D is often called the 'sunshine vitamin' because our bodies make it when our skin is exposed to sunlight. It helps keep bones, teeth, and muscles healthy. But in Ireland and the UK, sunshine isn't always reliable, especially during the long autumn and winter months. For adults, this means we sometimes need supplements, and for babies, it's even more important because their growing bodies are building strong bones from the very start.

Breastfed babies: Breast milk is wonderful and provides nearly everything your baby needs for the best start in life. But it doesn't contain enough vitamin D. Because of this, health experts recommend that all breastfed babies are given a daily vitamin D supplement in the form of drops from birth until they're one year old. Even if you or your partner are taking a vitamin D supplement yourself, babies still need their own drops.

Formula fed babies: Infant formula is different. By law, it

already has vitamin D added to it. This means that most formula-fed babies get enough without needing an extra supplement.

The important detail is how much formula your baby is drinking:

If your baby is having more than about 500ml (just under a pint) of formula a day, they're getting all the vitamin D they need from their feeds.

If they're having less than 500ml a day (for example, if you're combination feeding with both breast milk and formula), then a vitamin D supplement is still recommended.

Poop

All that black, tarry meconium will have cleared out of your baby's bowel by day three. The number of poopy nappies can vary from day to day and from baby to baby – at least one poop a day is common, but no need to panic if 24 hours go by without poop (unless your baby is presenting other symptoms).

In breastfed babies, the colour can vary, but it is usually yellowish. Texture-wise, breastfed poop is quite runny or watery and seedy – it is often compared to Dijon mustard. Formula-fed babies usually pass stools that have a similar colour and texture to peanut butter. (Apologies if this has turned you off mustard and peanut butter!)

Poop that is extremely pale, as in white or almost white, can be a sign of a rare problem with a baby's liver, so speak to your public-health nurse or GP if you notice this. If your baby does have this problem, their urine will also be a very dark, almost brown, colour.

Pee

What on earth are those orange or pink spots in my baby's pee? These are normal in the first few days and are due to tiny crystals in the urine called pyruvate crystals. As your baby's urine becomes more dilute, these spots should disappear. If they are still present after week one, speak to your public-health nurse or GP.

After day two or three, your baby's pee will vary from light to dark yellow, and they will have more and more wet nappies as the first week goes by. By day five or six, your baby will be having about six wet nappies a day. If your baby is still only having two or three wet nappies a day, they may not be getting enough to drink, so speak to your public-health nurse or GP.

Newborn pee doesn't usually have a strong smell, so if you do notice a strong or foul smell from the urine, speak to your public-health nurse or GP. Similarly, peeing should be effortless. If your baby is distressed or uncomfortable when peeing, they should be checked out by a healthcare professional.

Sleep

Your baby will be asleep more than awake in the first week. On average, your baby will sleep 18 to 19 hours per day. It might be hard for you to believe that they are only awake for a total of five or six hours; this is because they often sleep in short bursts known as 'sleep cycles', which last from 20 to 50 minutes. In the first few weeks, they will wake as often during the night as they do during the day, sometimes even more often.

There are also different types of sleep during these cycles. During active sleep, your baby might stretch or move, open their eyes, or cry a little. During quiet sleep, they will lie still and breathe quietly and regularly. Neither type of sleep is better than the other. Your baby is getting a good rest while they are asleep (even if you are not!).

When your newborn baby is awake, there are feeds and nappies and changes of clothes to be taken care of but, increasingly, your baby will seek out your face and interact with you for brief periods.

If your baby seems excessively sleepy or tired in the first week, if they are not waking for feeds, or seem too drowsy or tired to interact with you for brief periods, this can be a sign that they are not feeding enough or that they are unwell, so do speak to your GP or public-health nurse if this is the case.

Crying

Crying is a newborn's main means of communication. They use it to signal hunger, discomfort, a dirty nappy, tiredness – everything! In the first week, however, babies tend not to cry as much as they do when they get a little older.

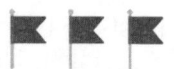

Crying is very normal, but non-stop crying, inconsolable crying, or sustained high-pitched crying is not. If your baby is crying like this in the first week of life, it could be a sign of irritability, which can happen if your baby is unwell. If you are concerned about your baby's crying, speak to your public-health nurse or GP.

Skin

Jaundice

Is it just me or is my baby turning yellow?

Well, yes, your baby might be turning yellow, and this is probably due to newborn jaundice, which is very common in the first week of life. It is more obvious in babies with lighter-coloured skin, but it can affect babies with all skin colours. In black- or brown-skinned babies, the main sign of jaundice can be yellowing of the whites of the eyes.

Jaundice is caused by a build-up of a chemical called bilirubin. It usually starts to improve after week two, as the liver becomes better at clearing bilirubin out of the bloodstream.

Contact your GP or public-health nurse if you notice jaundice in your baby. They may simply monitor your baby, send them for blood tests, or advise you to go to hospital. If the levels of bilirubin in the blood go over a certain level, your baby will need to be admitted for phototherapy. This involves placing your baby on a special blanket that emits a type of blue-green light, which breaks down the bilirubin in the skin. It usually takes a day or two of this treatment for the bilirubin levels to start to fall.

Rashes

My baby is covered in red spots!

This can look alarming, but it is unlikely to be serious. If your baby does develop a red bumpy rash, they should be reviewed by your GP or public-health nurse, but they are most likely going to reassure you that it is either baby acne or erythema toxicum.

Erythema toxicum sounds especially alarming, but it is a common and innocent rash in babies. It consists of areas of redness and sometimes fluid-filled blisters. Baby acne is slightly different, with red bumps, some of them developing into little pustules.

No treatment is required for either of these rashes.

Umbilical cord

How do I manage the umbilical cord stump?

The umbilical cord starts off plump, with a jelly-like texture but, when your baby is outside the womb, it starts to dry up. At birth, the cord is usually clamped with a plastic clip, and your baby will come home with their cord stump and this plastic clip attached. The stump usually shrivels up and falls off between days 5 and 15, but, until then, you will have to keep an eye on it to make sure that the skin around the base of the stump on your baby's tummy is clean, dry, and free of infection.

Inspect the stump at every nappy change – though you should wash your hands carefully before and after touching it. Make sure the skin looks clean and is the same colour as the skin on the rest of the tummy. Keep the top of the nappy folded down to avoid putting pressure on the stump.

If you notice the skin around the base of the cord turning red, ask your GP or public-health nurse to check your baby to rule out a skin infection.

Normal healing versus signs of infection

During normal healing, the stump may:

- turn from yellow-green to brown or black before falling off
- have a small amount of dried blood or clear discharge
- cause no discomfort to your baby.

However, you should contact your GP, public-health nurse, or out-of-hours doctor if you notice any of the following signs of infection:

- Redness spreading from the stump: A small rim of redness is common, but if the skin around the stump becomes increasingly red, warm, or swollen, this could indicate an infection.

- Pus or cloudy discharge: A small amount of clear or light-yellow fluid is normal, but thick, yellow-green, or foul-smelling pus is not.
- Bad odour: While the stump can have a mild smell as it dries, a strong, unpleasant odour can signal infection.
- Tenderness or swelling: If your baby seems in pain when the area is touched or the belly around the stump looks swollen, it's worth getting checked.
- Fever or general unwellness: Fever (temperature above 38°C), poor feeding, unusual sleepiness, or excessive crying could mean an infection is spreading and needs urgent attention.

CHECKING BABY'S TEMPERATURE

How can you tell if your baby has a fever? Or if they have an abnormally low temperature? When your baby is very young, even small changes in temperature can signal that something isn't quite right. Knowing how to take their temperature accurately is an important skill for parents. Here's what you need to know about the different methods available, how reliable they are, and which thermometers are recommended.

Can you tell by touch?

Many parents instinctively feel their baby's forehead, neck or back to check if they seem hot or cold. While touch is useful for spotting if your baby feels unusually warm, it is not a reliable way to detect fever. Hand-feel can easily miss a raised temperature or overestimate it if the baby is warm from clothes or blankets.

Recommended method

Touching your baby's skin can alert you that something's different, but it cannot replace a thermometer. For newborns, the safest and most accurate way of checking temperature is a digital thermometer under the armpit (known as the axillary method).

How to use: Place under the baby's armpit, ensuring good skin contact.

Pros: Accurate, safe, affordable, widely available.
Cons: Requires holding baby's arm still for a short time.

A reading of 38°C or more means that your baby has a fever. A reading of under 36°C means your baby's temperature is abnormally low.

Tips for taking a baby's temperature

Always follow the thermometer's instructions.

- Check the thermometer is clean before and after use.
- For an armpit reading, ensure the probe touches skin, not clothing.
- Take two readings if unsure and use the higher one.

If your baby has a fever, or an abnormally low temperature, is unusually sleepy, feeding poorly, or you're worried, always seek medical advice straight away.

Because the first week is when undiagnosed heart and metabolic conditions, or newborn sepsis can present, any sudden or concerning changes in your baby's behaviour (irritability), muscle tone (e.g. if they seem suddenly floppy) or temperature (either feeling cold to the touch or developing a fever) warrant urgent medical review and you should bring them to the local emergency department. We'd much prefer to see you there and reassure you all is well than have you wait at home with a potentially very unwell baby.

Facial appearance and head shape

Of course, every newborn baby is beautiful and perfect. But after the adrenaline and hormone rush of the first 24 hours wears off you may find yourself looking at your baby and wondering if everything is as it should be. You might notice that their head shape looks a little strange, or they have marks or bruises on their face or scalp. Or their eyes may appear bloodshot.

Why does a newborn's head look different?

During birth, your baby passes through the birth canal, a tight and pressurised journey. To make this possible, the bones of a baby's skull are not yet fused; they are soft and flexible, with small gaps called fontanelles (the 'soft spots'). This means the head can temporarily change shape to help your baby be born safely.

Common appearances include:

Elongated head: A temporary narrowing and lengthening of the skull after vaginal birth.
Flat areas: Pressure during delivery may cause mild flattening in places.
Asymmetry: One side may look different from the other for a short time.
Moulding lines: Subtle ridges where skull bones overlap during delivery.

These changes are usually short-lived and improve in the first few days to weeks of life. Babies born by caesarean section tend to be born with rounder heads at birth, as they haven't had such a tight squeeze on the way out of the womb!

Here are some other things you may notice about your baby's appearance.

Red eyes

The whites of your baby's eyes may appear bloodshot or red. This is known as a subconjunctival haemorrhage. It sounds dramatic, but it is simply due to the breakage of small blood vessels in the eyes of a baby. It does not harm the eye, and the redness will disappear in 7–10 days.

Bruising, swelling, and forceps/ventouse marks

If your baby's birth involved assistance, such as forceps or ventouse (vacuum) delivery, you may see:

- small marks or swelling where the instruments were used
- temporary puffiness of the face or scalp
- a soft swelling called a caput succedaneum or a firmer bump called a cephalohaematoma (a collection of blood under the scalp).

These usually heal without treatment over days to weeks.

When to seek advice

Most changes are harmless and improve naturally, but you should speak to your midwife, GP, or public-health nurse if you notice:

- swelling that seems to be getting worse, not better
- redness, warmth, or signs of infection
- persistent flattening on one side of the head after several weeks (positional plagiocephaly)
- concerns about your baby's development or comfort.

Birthmarks

There are four main types of birthmarks that you might notice during the first week.

The first, known as a 'stork bite' or an 'angel's kiss', is very common. It is an area of redness on the forehead, eyelids, nose, upper lip, or back of the neck, though it can look darker when the baby is crying or hot. The medical term for a stork bite is 'nevus simplex' and it occurs in almost one in every three babies. These stork bites are not serious and most disappear as your baby grows older.

Strawberry birthmarks, also known as 'strawberry naevi' or 'infantile haemangiomas', can appear as a little raised red dot in the first week or two after birth. They usually grow bigger over the first 6 to 12 months and then start to shrink, disappearing fully by around age two. These generally do not need any treatment, unless they are around the eyes, nose, mouth, or in the nappy area.

Blue-grey spots (previously called 'Mongolian blue spots') are also common, especially in babies with brown or black skin. They can look like a bruise and are usually found on the lower back, bottom, arms, or legs. These marks do not need any treatment and usually disappear fully by age four.

Port-wine stains ('nevus flammeus') are not common, affecting about 3 in every 1,000 babies. These birthmarks are darker than stork marks and can occur anywhere on the body and may cause cosmetic concerns for children if they are on the face. They do not fade with time, but laser treatment can reduce them significantly. Port-wine stains are not harmful, but if one is present on the upper part of your baby's face or the eyelid, it may mean another medical condition is present, so your baby should be referred for review by a paediatrician.

The weird stuff!

Have you heard of 'witch's milk'? The medical term is 'neonatal galactorrhoea' and it describes the secretion of milk from baby's nipples. It can affect girls *and* boys. Although it is not common, it is also not abnormal. It is a response of baby's breast tissue to maternal hormones, which cross the placenta in the womb. It should stop by about four weeks of age but if it does not stop, ask your GP to check your baby.

Another condition caused by exposure to maternal hormones in the womb is 'baby periods', which only affects girls. 'Baby periods' consist of minor vaginal bleeding in newborn girls, caused by the sudden drop-off in the mother's oestrogen after birth. The discharge is usually blood-tinged or pink, and it only lasts three to four days.

And something you might not have been expecting: was your baby born with teeth? These are called 'natal teeth'. Natal teeth are teeth that are present at birth or appear within the first month of life. They're uncommon, occurring in about one in every 2,000–3,000 babies, and usually show up in the lower front gums. While they may look surprising, natal teeth are often just part of the normal set of baby teeth that have erupted earlier than expected. Some are firm and harmless, but others may be small, loose, or sharp. This can sometimes cause problems like difficulty with breastfeeding, irritation of the baby's tongue, or, in rare cases, a risk of the tooth becoming loose enough to pose a choking hazard. If you notice a tooth in your newborn's mouth, point it out in the maternity hospital during your baby's check-up, or to your public-health nurse. The tooth can usually be safely left in place and just monitored, but if it causes feeding issues or is too loose, a dentist may recommend smoothing the tooth or removing it. The good news is that natal teeth are usually not a sign of anything serious.

Newborn screening tests

All babies will have a thorough physical examination within the first 72 hours after birth. This includes:

- a hip check to assess for hip dysplasia
- eye screening
- a heart exam
- a testicular exam in boys.

The newborn hearing screening is offered before discharge for babies born in hospital, or as an outpatient appointment for babies born at home.

The newborn heel prick (or blood spot) test is offered between days three and five. It checks for nine serious but rare conditions. There are huge benefits to diagnosing these conditions shortly after birth, because of the treatment and management plans that can be put in place. These conditions are:

Condition	What it means	If not picked up early	How screening helps your baby
Cystic fibrosis (CF)	A genetic condition that makes the body produce thick, sticky mucus, mainly affecting the lungs and digestion.	Chest infections, difficulty gaining weight, and shorter life expectancy.	Early care with medicines, physiotherapy, and nutrition helps children stay healthier and live longer.

36 | SHOULD I BE WORRIED?

Condition	What it means	If not picked up early	How screening helps your baby
Congenital hypothyroidism (CHT)	The thyroid gland doesn't make enough thyroid hormone, which is needed for growth and brain development.	Without treatment, babies may develop slow growth, learning difficulties, and delays.	A simple daily thyroid hormone medicine helps babies grow and develop normally.
Phenylketonuria (PKU)	Babies cannot break down a substance called phenylalanine found in food and drink.	Harmful build-up can cause brain damage, learning difficulties, and seizures.	A special low-protein diet and regular monitoring protect your child's development.
Classical galactosaemia (C Gal)	Babies cannot process galactose, a sugar in milk (including breast and formula milk).	Can cause feeding problems, liver damage, infections, and long-term health issues.	Removing galactose from the diet straight away prevents life-threatening illness.
Glutaric aciduria type 1 (GA1)	Babies have difficulty breaking down certain proteins.	Illness or fasting can trigger brain injury, leading to movement and co-ordination problems.	A special diet and emergency treatment during illness reduce the risk of harm.
Medium-chain acyl-CoA dehydrogenase deficiency (MCADD)	The body cannot use some fats for energy when a baby is unwell or hasn't eaten for a while.	Can cause very low blood sugar, seizures, coma, or sudden death.	Avoiding long fasting and giving glucose when ill keeps babies safe and well.
Homocystinuria (HCU)	Babies cannot properly process an amino acid called methionine.	Can cause eye problems, blood clots, learning difficulties, and bone problems.	A special diet, vitamins, and medicines help reduce risks and protect health.

Condition	What it means	If not picked up early	How screening helps your baby
Maple syrup urine disease (MSUD)	Babies cannot break down certain proteins in food. Urine may smell sweet, like maple syrup.	Build-up of harmful substances can cause brain swelling, seizures, coma, or death.	A special diet and close medical monitoring prevent serious illness.
Adenosine deaminase deficiency severe combined immunodeficiency (ADA-SCID)	A rare condition where the immune system doesn't work, leaving babies unable to fight infections.	Life-threatening infections usually start within the first year of life.	Early treatment (such as a stem cell transplant, gene therapy, or enzyme treatment) can give babies the chance to grow up healthy.

Hip dysplasia

Developmental dysplasia of the hip (DDH) is something all newborns are screened for in Ireland.

In some babies, the ball-and-socket joint of the hip doesn't form quite as it should. The socket might be shallow or the ball might be a little loose. Left untreated, it can cause problems with walking later in childhood.

How is it screened for?

Every baby in Ireland has their hips checked by a doctor or midwife within the first couple of days after birth. They gently move your baby's legs to feel for any looseness or 'clicks'.

Some babies need a follow-up ultrasound scan of the hips. This is especially likely if:

- they were breech at birth
- there's a family history of DDH
- there are concerns from the first examination.

The scan is quick, painless and usually done around four to six weeks of age.

Why early detection matters

The earlier DDH is found, the easier it is to fix – and the less likely it will cause trouble later. If DDH is spotted during the hip check, your baby might be given a soft harness (often called a 'Pavlik harness') to keep their hips in the best position for growth. This is worn for several weeks, and most little ones adapt to it without fuss.

Follow-up care

If your baby is diagnosed with DDH, you'll be referred to a children's orthopaedic team. They'll keep a close eye on your baby's progress, with regular check-ups and repeat scans or X-rays as needed. The length of follow-up varies, but some children are monitored until they're walking confidently.

Physiotherapists often play a role too, especially after the harness treatment ends. Physios can provide guidance on gentle stretches, exercises, and safe ways to carry and position your baby to support strong, healthy hips.

If you're told your baby needs a scan or a harness, try not to panic. With prompt treatment, the vast majority of children go on to run, jump, and dance without any hip problems at all.

CAR SEATS

If you had your baby in hospital, then you need to have a plan for getting your baby home. And that plan will always involve a car seat. It's the law that your baby must travel in a properly fitted car seat from the very first journey home.

Choosing a car seat for your newborn can feel a little overwhelming, but it's really about keeping your baby safe and comfortable on every journey. For the first stage, you'll need a rear-facing infant car seat that is the right size for your baby's weight and height – most are suitable from birth. Always follow the manufacturer's instructions when fitting the seat, making sure the harness is snug and the seat is firmly secured in your car. Whatever you do, don't let the first time you try out the car seat be the day you are leaving the hospital with the baby in the car seat! Many local shops, baby stores, and road safety services in Ireland and the UK offer free fitting checks, so don't hesitate to ask for help to be sure everything is installed correctly. Taking the time to get it right will give you peace of mind and the best protection for your little one.

CONGRATULATIONS!

Your baby is now one week old. How are you doing? Check in with yourself. It has been a momentous week.

If this is your first baby, your world has changed entirely. You are learning to be a parent for the very first time, and your baby has just spent their very first week out in the world.

Over the next few weeks, even more change is to come, with your baby reaching all sorts of incredible milestones, including gorgeous gummy baby smiles.

If this is your second, third (or even beyond that) child, you are probably in the throes of marvelling at how different this baby is from their siblings. And their siblings are adjusting to becoming big brothers and sisters.

What an incredible seven days.

CHAPTER 2
2 to 6 Weeks

In these next few weeks, your baby will grow through the newborn stage. When you look back at the pictures and memories of the first few weeks, you will hardly believe how much has changed, not least how much your baby has grown. On average, babies gain about 1 kilogram and grow 3–4 centimetres in the first six weeks.

Their head circumference increases by 3–4 centimetres as well, reflecting brain growth. With that growing brain comes developmental milestones, and you will see lots of those in the first six weeks. So, let's delve into all of the amazing changes that you are about to see in your baby.

FEEDING

Whether your baby is breastfed or bottle fed, over the first six weeks you will learn to recognise when your baby is hungry. Even though they can't talk, they will have a 'hungry cry'. Before they get to the crying stage, they will have more subtle cues that you will quickly become an expert at spotting. Their hands might come to their face or mouth, they may smack their lips and, if you stroke their cheek, they might turn their head and try to latch on to your finger. This is called 'rooting' and, aside from being a good indicator of hunger, it is super cute!

If you are breastfeeding, the first four weeks are the time where your milk supply becomes established, and you and your baby get into a feeding routine. These routines can vary between babies, with some babies taking regular, spaced-out feeds, and others clustering their feeds together at certain times of the day (or night!). Breastfed babies often wake several times during the night for feeds. There is no need to introduce a feeding schedule for breastfed babies; they are very good at setting the pace themselves, and you will quickly get to know their hunger pattern.

I had a very hard time establishing breastfeeding with my first baby, trying to get her to latch on. I foolishly thought that breastfeeding baby number two would be a walk in the park, but we encountered a whole different set of issues, with my milk taking forever to come in. Every baby is unique, as is every breastfeeding journey.

Having grown up being surrounded by bottle-fed siblings and cousins, the thing I found hardest about breastfeeding the first-time round was not knowing how much my baby was actually drinking. Because I could not get my baby to latch on for the first three weeks, I had to pump and feed. When I was doing this, I knew how much milk she was getting, but when I finally had a consultation with a lactation consultant, and we figured things out, I could put the pump away. Then, I became super nervous about the amount she was getting with each feed. But I gained confidence with every wet nappy and every gram my little one gained. She was having about six or seven wet nappies a day, indicating that she was getting enough fluids. I knew we were doing okay when the public-health nurse did an extra weight check at four weeks and she had gained 200 grams in a week.

If your baby is having issues latching on, or sucking and swallowing, or you are having nipple pain whilst feeding, it is important to speak to your GP practice nurse, public-health nurse or lactation consultant. Your baby might be referred for tongue-tie assessment or you might just need a few tips on how to best position your baby on the breast. Although breastfeeding is 'natural', it is not an innate skill. It is something that must be taught by people who are appropriately qualified.

If your baby is being bottle fed, either expressed breast milk (EBM) or formula (breast milk substitute), you will have a better idea how much milk they are getting over a 24-hour period.

Typically, by the second week, if you are pumping and feeding EBM, you will produce 500–700 millilitres over 24 hours, and feed this to your baby via bottle on demand. The amount of milk you produce will increase every week. A baby being fed on formula needs 150 millilitres of milk per kilogram over 24 hours. So, for example, a 5-kilogram baby will need 750 millilitres of milk over 24 hours (150 x 5 = 750), divided into six to eight feeds. It is no longer recommended to space these feeds out every three to four hours, but rather to respond to baby's hunger cues throughout the day (and night!).

No matter how your baby is fed, the main indicator that they are getting enough food is their weight gain. Some weight loss is normal in the first week after birth but, by week two, your baby should be back to their birth weight. From then on, they will gain 150–200 grams per week.

Your GP or GP practice nurse will check your baby's weight at two and six weeks. We used to use a horrible term if a baby was not gaining weight: 'failure to thrive'. Thankfully, we got rid of the word 'failure', because nobody is failing, least of all the baby and the parents! So now we refer to slower-than-expected weight gain as 'faltering growth'.

Faltering growth

There are a few reasons why your baby might not gain weight. I know from experience that this can be super stressful for parents, regardless of how your baby is fed. But let's break down the reasons and have a look at how some of them can be addressed.

Genetics

Some babies are born above the percentile where they will eventually settle, perhaps due to gestational diabetes or an efficient placenta that really delivers on those nutrients whilst in the womb. This essentially means some babies are born weighing more than average, but they will gradually drift towards average, or smaller than average, because their parents are average or smaller than average in size. As long as your baby is happy and feeding well, and they have good stores of fat visible on those adorable baby legs and arms, your GP or public-health nurse will probably just continue to monitor them and not request any extra tests or paediatrician reviews.

Babies with Down syndrome also have a different rate of growth throughout childhood, and your GP or public-health nurse will use a specific growth chart to track their weight and length.

Issues with latching on or supply

This issue relates to babies who are breastfeeding. The role of a lactation consultant cannot be emphasised enough here. They will monitor your baby for signs of tongue-tie and help you to assess and build your milk supply if needed.

Pain or discomfort when feeding

A baby who is experiencing pain when feeding will quickly learn to associate feeding with discomfort and may start to refuse feeds.

One cause of pain whilst feeding is oral thrush. This causes a white coating on the tongue and sometimes on the lips. If breastfeeding, the thrush may also affect your nipples, causing you pain when baby latches on. There is effective treatment for thrush, so, if you suspect your baby has it, do speak to your public-health nurse, GP practice nurse, or GP.

A more challenging cause of pain and discomfort on feeding

can be infant reflux. Posseting, which means bringing up a small amount of milk after feeds, occurs in almost all babies. The junction where the food pipe (oesophagus) meets the stomach usually closes after food (or milk) has gone into the stomach to prevent stomach contents travelling back up the food pipe. However, in babies, the muscles at this junction have not become fully functional, so it is normal for a little milk to travel back up the food pipe – and land on your shoulder! In some babies, however, the amounts of milk escaping the stomach are bigger, and the milk has been mixed with acid in the stomach, so it can cause a burning, uncomfortable sensation in the food pipe. Even tiny babies will quickly learn to associate feeding with this uncomfortable feeling, and might become fussy or irritable when placed on the breast or offered a bottle.

Signs of reflux in very young babies include frequent hiccupping, irritability during feeding, back arching during feeding, refusing to feed, and excessive spitting up of milk. Not all babies with reflux spit up, however. If you suspect reflux in your newborn, speak to your GP or public-health nurse.

Not enough energy

Calories provide energy. A baby needs to drink and absorb enough calories in order to gain weight and grow. Therefore, if they are either not drinking enough or not absorbing the nutrients well, they may not gain weight. A baby may have a poor milk intake due to poor latch-on or poor supply if breastfed, or pain or discomfort.

Your baby may be drinking enough milk to meet their calorie needs, but they may not be absorbing the nutrients well. This can happen if your baby is formula fed and has a cow's-milk-protein intolerance or allergy (CMPI/CMPA). This causes inflammation in the gut, which leads to diarrhoea and means the gut is unable to absorb the nutrition from the milk. This is the most common cause of poor absorption of nutrients in babies (known in medical terms as 'malabsorption'). Your baby will need to switch to a specialised formula, which is either extensively hydrolysed (broken down) or amino-acid based. Apart from CMPI/CMPA, there are other rare gut-malabsorption problems that need specialised assessment in order to be diagnosed.

If your baby has faltering growth, your public-health nurse or GP will examine your baby, ask you about how well they are feeding, and, if their rate of growth does not improve, possibly refer you to a specialised clinic or paediatrician for further tests. The important thing is not to feel bad or worry too much. Faltering growth in your baby is not your fault. Your doctor just needs to figure out what is going on and how to help your baby.

If a newborn baby becomes breathless during a feed and is unable to feed well as a result, this is a red flag. Sometimes, this breathlessness is also associated with excessive sweating. If you notice your baby becoming breathless and/or sweaty when feeding, speak to your GP immediately, as this can be a sign of an issue with baby's heart.

POOP

When you were expecting your baby, you probably had no idea how big a deal poop would become in your life. Why is it that colour? How can a baby poop that much? Why hasn't my baby pooped for days? The list goes on!

There is a difference in the poop of breastfed babies versus formula-fed babies, so let's start there.

Breastfed babies tend to have runnier poop that is yellowish in colour and has what looks like mustard seeds mixed through it. Normal colours in breastfed baby poop are yellow, brown and green. It hardly smells at all.

Most breastfed babies will poop up to five times a day, usually after a feed but, as the weeks go on, you might notice your baby does not poop as often, and some breastfed babies might go up to five days without a bowel motion. You will quickly learn what is normal for your baby, but a general guideline is that if your breastfed baby has not pooped for a week or more, you should speak to your GP.

You might notice blood in your breastfed baby's stool. If this is dark, it might have come from the mother's nipples during feeding, but if it is bright red, it is more likely to have come from your baby's bowel. If you notice blood in your baby's stool, speak to your GP.

Formula-fed babies' poop is a little different. It has a toothpaste consistency and a yellow to brown colour. Normal colours in formula-fed baby poop are yellow, brown and green, and formula-fed babies will usually have two to four dirty nappies over 24 hours.

You will quickly become familiar with your baby's poop pattern. If they are pooping a lot more or a lot less than usual, you should contact your GP.

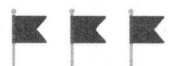

Regardless of whether your baby is breastfed or formula fed, you should seek medical attention if their poop is white or red.

Constipation

Constipation is the infrequent passing of dry, hard stools associated with straining and discomfort. It is rare in newborns, but it can happen. However, some babies can *seem* constipated –

grunting and straining and going very red – but passing normal-looking soft poops. So why all the distress in these babies?

Well, they may have an issue called 'infant dyschezia'. For a bowel motion to succeed, two things need to happen at the same time: the pelvic floor needs to relax and the tummy muscles need to contract. This takes co-ordination, so your baby needs to learn to poop. Until it clicks for them, they will cry, which tenses the tummy muscles, until by chance they manage to also relax their pelvic floor and, hey presto, a poop! The crying, grunting, and red-face episodes can last up to 30 minutes, and these episodes might go on for up to two weeks, but, eventually, your baby will get the hang of pooping. So, despite the serious-sounding name, infant dyschezia is actually a normal part of many babies' development, and they grow out of it.

However, if a baby is having episodes of grunting, straining and/or crying when trying to have a bowel motion, and they are passing small, hard stools, then they may well be constipated.

If your baby is formula fed and becomes constipated, check to make sure that the formula is being made up correctly and that your baby is getting the correct amount for their age and weight. Do not dilute the formula. Do not offer the baby bottles of cool boiled water without input from your GP, GP practice nurse, or public-health nurse. Babies under 6 months should not be given water because their little tummies can fill up quickly, leaving less room for the breast milk or formula they need for growth. Too much water can also upset the balance of salts in their blood, leading to 'water intoxication', which may cause seizures or other serious health problems.

A warm bath and gentle tummy massage may help baby's bowels to move. 'Bicycling' the legs by gently moving them up and down while baby is lying on their back may also help.

Your baby should be seen by a doctor for their constipation if it lasts more than two days or if any of the following occur:

- they are very distressed
- you feel very concerned
- they have a fever
- their appetite decreases
- they start to vomit
- their tummy is bloated or distended
- they develop bloody stools
- they stop gaining or start losing weight.

Usually there is nothing more complex going on when it comes to constipation, but in rare cases it can be a sign of an underlying condition. For example, Hirschsprung's disease is an abnormal nerve supply to the bowel, and babies with this condition are usually slow to pass meconium (the first black, tarry poo) after birth. An underactive thyroid can also cause constipation. In the past, cystic fibrosis would often present as severe constipation in newborns, but it is now screened for at birth in Ireland.

PEE

Peeing is usually straightforward for newborn babies. They will have between four and eight wet nappies a day, and the colour will be similar to an adult's pee. Pale yellow and frequent pees mean your baby is well hydrated; dark yellow and less frequent pees might be a sign of dehydration.

Red pee

In the first week, your baby may have passed pinkish pee. This colour is due to pyruvate crystals and should disappear as baby starts to drink more. If it persists, you will need to get your baby checked out.

Equally, if you notice blood in your baby girl's nappy, it may be normal (remember those newborn periods we talked about on page 34?), but it is not normal if it starts when they are over two weeks old, and it should not continue for more than three to four days. Blood in a little boy's pee is never normal. Bottom line, if you are seeing blood in your baby's nappy between the ages of two and six weeks old, you need to get them medically assessed.

Urinary tract infections

Urinary tract infections (UTIs) in newborns can be extremely serious, even life-threatening. They are more common in boys in this age group, but can also occur in girls, and they can be caused by a problem with the tubes that drain urine from the kidneys to the bladder. (In older age groups, UTIs are more common in girls. See page 187.)

As tiny babies cannot express how they are feeling, the signs of a UTI can be hard to spot early on. There can be some subtle clues, such as upset or discomfort whilst peeing or an unusual smell from the urine. The strength of flow of urine in baby boys is also important. Normally if a little boy pees with his nappy off, he's like a little fountain. A trickling or weak flow can be a sign of a blockage in the bladder. However, the most common signs of a UTI will be vomiting, fever, and irritability. Fever can be a late sign, so if your baby develops new vomiting that is forceful (as opposed to possetting or reflux), you will need to get them checked by a doctor.

Fever in any baby under three months old needs medical review, and the urine must always be checked for infection.

GENITALIA

'It's a girl!'

'It's a boy!'

These are amongst the first pronouncements made about your newborn baby, and it's usually pretty easy to tell which is which. We recognise and assign gender at birth based on the appearance of the external genitalia, i.e. the genitalia we can see on the outside.

Baby girls do not have much visible externally. The labia (those fleshy parts that cover up everything) can be somewhat swollen in the first few weeks due to exposure to maternal hormones in the womb.

The labia should be easy to separate and not fused together. This will be checked during the newborn physical exam, as well as making sure that the tube that comes from the bladder (urethra) is open and allowing urine to pass.

When cleaning newborn girls' genitalia, very gently pass a wet cotton ball or baby wipe between the labia from front to back. This is to avoid transferring bacteria from poop at the back up towards the front, where the urethra opens to the surface. If that happens, it can lead to a UTI. Sometimes, as the maternal hormones leave the baby's body, the labia can start to fuse together. If you notice this, speak to your GP or public-health nurse.

Baby boys have more visible genitalia. The scrotum contains the testicles and, at birth, the scrotum can seem very swollen due to the influence of maternal hormones. The swelling can make it hard to feel if the testicles are in the scrotum, but this will be checked as part of the newborn exam. If the testicles have not descended into the scrotum at birth, this will need to be monitored. If the testicles have not moved into the scrotum by six months of age, they are unlikely to do so without surgical assistance. The procedure is called an orchidopexy and is usually performed between the ages of one and two. It is important to move the testicles into the scrotum as they need to grow and develop in the slightly lower temperature there in order to avoid problems with fertility and an increased risk of testicular cancer in adult life.

Your baby boy's penis will measure about 3.5 centimetres. At the tip of the penis, you will find the foreskin. When cleaning a baby boy's genitalia, there is no need to pull back the foreskin to clean the penis. At this age, the foreskin is too tight to be retractable and will not be retractable until they are over the age of five. Simply wash the area gently with water.

The penis can become erect in baby boys. This is especially common when they are about to pee. It is normal and there is no need to worry about it.

In rare cases, in both baby boys and girls, it is not so easy to tell the gender from looking at the genitalia. A very small number of babies are born with external genitalia that do not look typical for their gender. This is known as having 'atypical genitalia'. These babies need specialised care and investigations, including ultrasound scans, and hormonal and genetic testing.

DEVELOPMENTAL MILESTONES

Your baby's brain and body develop so much in the first six weeks. As your baby gets bigger, they learn how to hold their head up without support, their vision develops, and their little eyes will learn to follow you as you move. One magical day, their face will light up with a little gummy smile that is for you, not because they have wind!

The word 'milestones' fills some parents with dread. Let's be real – you are going to meet some competitive parents who seem to think reaching milestones is some sort of race. The healthcare professionals who check your baby do not see things like this, and there are no prizes handed out to the baby who walks first! Instead, we use developmental milestones as a tool to detect signs of possible neurodevelopmental issues, so that interventions and assistance can be introduced early if needed. We also bear in mind that all babies develop differently, so please don't worry too much if a healthcare professional flags your baby as being a little behind in meeting a milestone.

By six weeks, the developmental milestones that will be checked for in your baby are grouped into four categories:

- gross motor: the big movements of the neck, trunk, arms, and legs
- fine motor and vision: smaller movements of the hands and fingers, reaching for objects, how well the eyes focus on faces and objects
- communication and hearing
- social and emotional.

Most babies born at full-term will have met milestones in all of these categories by six weeks.

Gross motor skills

Your six-week-old is probably able to lift up their head briefly when placed on their tummy. When you hold them in your arms, they can probably hold their head up independently. When lying on their back, they should be able to lift their arms and legs and kick their legs.

Fine motor skills and vision

Your baby may attempt to reach out for objects dangling in front of their face. In order to do this, they need to be able to see. At six weeks, most babies can focus on a bright object and track its movement with their eyes – a skill known as 'fixing and following'. Your baby can usually follow you with their eyes as you move around the room. By six weeks, most babies will seek eye contact with their caregivers.

Communication and hearing

By the time your baby is six weeks old, they will turn their head towards the source of a sound, particularly if that sound is a familiar voice. They will also probably still have an involuntary startle response to loud noises. Your baby will also be starting to make sounds of their own outside of crying. They may make cooing sounds, and you may find yourself having a back-and-forth 'chat' with your baby as they coo in response to your voice.

Social and emotional milestones

The big social and emotional milestone that most babies have met at six weeks is the social smile. This is a smile that is in response to your voice or facial expressions. It is very hard to explain the happiness that your baby's first smile will bring. Just make sure to enjoy the moment.

SLEEP

One of the things you can never be truly prepared for, especially as a first-time parent, is how your sleep patterns are going to change. Here is this tiny being, dependent on you to tend to their every need, at any hour of the day or night. In the first six weeks, your baby does not have a circadian rhythm. That is to say, their brain cannot tell the difference between day and night. In general, their pattern is eat, pee, poop, sleep, repeat.

Sleep usually comes in two- to four-hour chunks, and this does not alter depending on the time of day. As your baby becomes more alert and engaged, you are as likely to have cooing and smiles at 1 am as you are at 1 pm. And that is going to play havoc with *your* circadian rhythm. It will not be forever, but that is cold comfort at 3 am on a Friday morning. From about eight weeks, however, your baby will start to learn the difference between day and night, so the nighttime wakings may become shorter, meaning they may sleep for slightly longer stretches at night.

If your baby is gaining weight and feeding well, you don't need to wake them for a night feed. Some parents like the idea of a 'dream feed'. This is a personal choice and involves lifting your sleeping baby for a feed, without fully waking them, just before you go to bed yourself. This is done in the hope that the baby's sleeping time can be stretched out so that you might manage to have a good sleep too. It is important not to force a dream feed, and you should always burp the baby and hold them upright, usually over the shoulder, for about 10 minutes after feeding.

Where should my baby sleep?

For the first six months, your baby should sleep in your room, but in a separate crib or cot. Remember ABC: **a**lone, on their **b**ack, in their **c**ot. This is the safest option to prevent potential injury and sudden infant death syndrome (SIDS, see page 360).

When you first start to consider where your baby might sleep, you will probably be on the receiving end of a barrage of advertising about the latest cot or crib, with a dizzying array of features like rocking and white-noise or 'fashionable' aesthetics. But is any of it necessary? In short, no. A firm, flat sleep surface, such as a bedside crib, is perfectly safe and adequate for the first three to four months. Just make sure that whatever you choose has a well-fitting mattress. Bedding should consist of a snugly fitted sheet, and either a sleep sack appropriate for your baby's weight or a cellular blanket.

Pillows, positioning nests, duvets, and cot bumpers are not only unnecessary, but also unsafe. Pillows and positioning nests can push a baby's chin onto their chest, which can lead to an unsafe sleep position known as 'chin to chest'. The reason this is unsafe is that a baby's airway is smaller than your little finger, and when their chin rests on their chest, it can cause their tiny airway to become kinked and blocked, resulting in a life-threatening situation known as 'positional asphyxia'. This means that baby cannot breathe.

Duvets and cot bumpers can cover a baby's face. Babies are sensitive to the levels of carbon dioxide in the air. If their face is covered by a duvet or if their face is buried in a bumper, they will end up breathing back in the air they just exhaled, which is high in carbon dioxide. This results in a phenomenon known as 'rebreathing', which is thought to increase the risk of SIDS.

The Lullaby Trust is a UK-based charity that spearheaded the Back to Sleep campaign in 1991, which has had the single biggest impact on reducing the number of babies dying from SIDS. They advise against bed-sharing, but acknowledge that some parents will end up bed-sharing with their babies.

According to their guidelines:

- The safest place for a baby to sleep is in a separate cot or Moses basket in the same room as their parents for the first six months.
- Bed-sharing increases the risk of SIDS if parents smoke, have consumed alcohol or drugs, are extremely tired, or if the baby was born prematurely or with a low birth weight.
- If parents choose to bed-share, they should ensure the baby is on their back on a firm, flat mattress with no pillows, duvets, or soft bedding around them.
- Sleeping with your baby on a sofa or armchair is extremely dangerous and should always be avoided.

BABYWEARING OR USING A BABY CARRIER

You might find using a baby sling or carrier very useful and practical. It enables you to keep your baby close, whilst having your hands free. However, it is extremely important to use these safely because if your newborn slouches down in the sling or carrier, they may get into an unsafe position that makes it hard for them to breathe, which can lead to 'positional asphyxia'.

Thankfully, there are now clear guidelines for parents to help them use baby slings and carriers safely. These are called the TICKS rules for safe babywearing, a guideline developed by the UK Sling Consortium. These rules are now widely recognised by health professionals and babywearing educators.

TICKS

T – Tight
The carrier should be tight, with your baby held close against you. Loose slings can cause your baby to slump, which can restrict breathing. A snug fit also supports your back and keeps your baby in a stable position.

I – In View at All Times
You should always be able to see your baby's face by simply glancing down. The fabric of the sling or carrier should never cover your baby's face.

C – Close Enough to Kiss
Your baby should be high enough on your chest that you can easily kiss the top of their head. If you have to bend your head down or move fabric out of the way, they're likely too low.

K – Keep Chin Off the Chest
Babies must not be curled so that their chin is forced onto their chest, which can restrict breathing. There should always be at least a finger's-width space under your baby's chin.

S – Supported Back
Your baby's back should be supported in a natural position, with their tummy and chest against you. Make sure the carrier holds your baby in a way that keeps their spine in alignment and hips in a healthy, seated 'M' position.

As well as the TICKS rules, here are some extra tips for safe babywearing:

- Layer wisely: With Ireland's changeable weather, it's tempting to overdress babies in a sling. Remember, your body heat adds warmth. Dress your baby in one layer fewer than you'd use in a pram and monitor them for overheating by checking how warm their chest or tummy feels.
- Avoid bulk: Avoid padded snowsuits inside a carrier – they can affect positioning and make it harder to judge your baby's temperature.
- Practise over a bed or sofa: If you're trying a new sling or learning to position baby, do so over a soft surface, ideally with help the first few times.
- Check local babywearing libraries: There are excellent sling libraries across Ireland and the UK offering support and carrier loans. They're a brilliant resource for finding the right fit.

Babywearing is wonderful when done safely. It can help babies settle, support breastfeeding, and make parenting life more manageable. By following the TICKS rules, you're helping to ensure that your baby is not only close and comforted, but safe.

For more support, ask your public-health nurse, GP, or a local sling consultant (search online for consultants in your area). They're there to help.

CRYING AND COLIC

Between weeks two and six, your baby might start to display more signs of fussiness, crying, or colic – and this can be a real shock to the system.

Colic is defined as crying for more than three hours a day, more than three days a week, for more than three weeks – a neat clinical definition that utterly fails to encapsulate the stress and anxiety that colic can cause parents.

In addition to crying, a baby with colic may exhibit other symptoms, such as restlessness, drawing up their legs, and finding it very hard to settle.

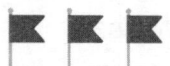

A baby who has started to cry more than they used to or is very hard to settle needs to be medically reviewed, and there are some important red flags to check for in a crying baby. These include:

- a weak or high-pitched cry
- a change in how the cry sounds
- poor feeding
- not gaining weight
- a distended or bloated tummy
- vomiting
- fever
- parental concern.

One thing that is extremely important to remember at all times when dealing with a baby who cries a lot and has a diagnosis of colic is that if you ever feel like you might respond in a way that could harm you or your baby, you need to ask for help immediately. If you are feeling extremely stressed and no one is available to watch your baby, make sure that your baby is safe (e.g. put them in their cot), go into another room, and take a breather. A short period of being in another room while your baby cries will not harm your baby and may help you a lot.

There is a huge overlap between parental mental-health issues and colic. Up to 25% of parents, both mums and dads, will have post-partum mental-health issues, including depression and anxiety; up to 20% of babies will have colic. This means there are a lot of households in which both parents and babies are struggling.

The online space makes getting through colic even more difficult. On social media, there is relentless messaging that parents should feel happy and blessed, yet a quick internet search will find you bombarded with products and treatments that promise to 'cure' your baby's colic.

Unfortunately, there is no quick fix for colic, but there are lots of things you can do to help your baby. It is okay to hold your baby to comfort them. The idea that a newborn might somehow be spoiled by being held and soothed is outdated and harmful. However, whilst this may help some babies with colic, other babies prefer to be laid down in a safe environment and not handled too much when they are upset. You will figure out which your baby prefers.

Winding your baby during and after feeds can be helpful if the crying is triggered by tummy discomfort. A warm bath can also sometimes help, as can baby massage. Some babies are soothed by motion, such as being taken for a walk in their buggy or a drive in the car, and some babies find white noise comforting.

Looking after yourself is extremely important during this time. It's okay to acknowledge your own feelings. Equally, it's important to remember that it's not your fault that your baby has colic, and your baby's crying is not a rejection of you as a parent. Please reach out to friends, family, other parents, your doctor, or your public-health nurse if you are struggling.

The crying will eventually resolve as your baby gets older, but it is okay to ask for help along the way. (I have also covered colic, including PURPLE crying, on page 317.)

MY STORY

I thought it might be helpful to write about my own experience of colic with my first child, so that, if you are going through it, you will know that you are not alone, that there is help available, and that it does end.

My first baby was easily the most beautiful baby to ever arrive on Earth (so is every baby – oxytocin is a wonderful hormone!). For the first few weeks, she, her dad, and I existed in the most amazing love bubble. Her dad was off work on paternity leave, I had support from my own family, and everything was just warm and cosy and wonderful.

Then, everyone else went back to their 'normal' life and it was just me and the baby at home all day until her dad arrived home from work. And a pattern started to emerge: about 30 minutes before her dad arrived home, the baby would start to cry. It would start as a little fussiness but, by the time he turned the key in the front door, she would be in a full-throated wail, with me frantically shushing her. He would offer to take her, I would refuse, somehow believing that this was a test of my skills as a mother and handing her over while she was crying would be some sort of failure on my part. I was not thinking clearly. My sole focus was to stop the crying and restore my baby's happiness.

I had a difficult pregnancy, especially in the final few weeks, so, after the baby was born, I was hypervigilant, even though I was completely exhausted. When the baby wasn't crying, I compulsively checked her to make sure she was still breathing. I hardly slept.

Looking back, I must have had some sort of post-natal anxiety, but there wasn't much awareness of that issue back when I had my first. I had done all the reading on parenting a newborn and, again – damagingly – back in those days, there was a philosophy that a baby should only be held when being fed, winded, changed, or bathed – as if the baby had some sort of corruptible hard drive and holding her close would somehow instil 'bad habits'.

When colic came to our home, I longed to hold my baby, and I'm sure she longed to be held. But I hovered at the end of the Moses basket, aching to hold her, filling the air with my cries too, trying to follow the advice I had read, feeling like a terrible mother.

We were living in a city far from both sides of the family. My husband and I felt desperately alone as we tried to figure out this tiny ball of human anguish. The days felt like months. The weeks felt like years. If she was crying, we were stressed. If she was not crying, we were stressed that she was about to start crying. When you are that tired and that stressed, you are just scrabbling around at the bottom of a dark hole, and you don't have the headspace to figure out your escape. Your internal resourcefulness is gone. You need help. Crucially, you need to *ask* for help.

For me, the help came from two places. First, my GP was incredibly kind and sympathetic. He gave me the reassurance I needed that my baby was okay and that I wasn't doing anything wrong. The second source of help came from a mum I had connected with in an online parenting forum, who had become my friend in real life. She had danced the colic dance too and encouraged me to hold and soothe my baby. I started using a baby carrier (see page 55 for how to do this safely), which made an instant difference for me and my little girl. We both had the connection we had clearly been longing for, and I subconsciously gave myself permission to follow my own instincts when parenting my baby. I don't think that that mum will ever realise how much she helped me with her honesty about her own struggles, her listening ear, and her non-judgemental advice.

My baby still screamed her little lungs out when she got tired or overstimulated, but I gradually became more attuned to her language, to what she was telling me. I loved her from the very start, but it took me three months to understand her.

Colic is different for every baby and every parent, and these are the things that helped me and my baby. What works for you and for your baby won't necessarily be the same.

My advice as a mum who has been there with colic is this:

- Forget about being the 'perfect' parent. Ignore the social-media posts about those 'dream babies'.
- Tune out from those who say 'it will pass'. Yes, it will pass, but right now you are suffering and your baby is upset. What you need is love and support.
- Come up for air if you can. Take the focus off your baby for one minute and ask yourself, 'How am I doing?' The answer may well be, 'Not great.' And if that is your answer, ask for help.

ILLNESS

There is no sugar-coating this: if your baby has a fever (38°C or above) in the first three months of life, they need to be medically reviewed and will likely be sent to the emergency department for assessment.

Why?

A fever almost always means your baby has a viral or bacterial infection and, because of their immature immune systems, they are at risk of serious illness if they get an infection. A baby under three months old must be assessed for infection and carefully observed. Babies in this age group are at higher risk of sepsis, meningitis, and pneumonia.

Fever may be the first (and sometimes only) sign that your baby is seriously unwell. If you do get sent to the emergency department because your baby has a fever, they will most likely do blood tests, urine tests, and viral swabs in the hospital. They may also perform a lumbar puncture if they cannot identify the source of the infection. It can be very scary to have to go through this with your baby, but not thoroughly assessing a newborn with a fever can have terrible consequences for their health.

A baby under three months old with a temperature of 38°C or above needs to be medically reviewed. Take them to see your GP or the out-of-hours GP service if you have access to one. If you cannot get an appointment with a GP, go to the emergency department.

Aside from a fever, there are other signs that your baby may be unwell. If you notice any of the following, then your baby needs to be seen by a doctor:

- **Excessive fussiness:** Your baby may be impossible to console and their cry may have a different tone to usual. For example, it may sound high-pitched.
- **Bulging fontanelle:** The soft spot at the top of your baby's head is usually level with the rest of their scalp. If the skin over the soft spot starts to bulge upwards, it can be a sign of raised pressure around the brain, so your baby will need to be medically assessed.
- **Signs of dehydration:** When your baby is dehydrated, either due to reduced fluid intake or increased loss through vomiting or diarrhoea, they may have fewer wet nappies, less tear production, and a sunken fontanelle.
- **Excessive sleepiness:** Your baby may be sleeping more than normal or not waking for feeds as normal. Excessive sleepiness may mean decreased consciousness, which is a sign of serious illness.
- **Vomiting:** You will be used to your baby spitting up small amounts of milk after feeds. This posseting is normal and effortless, while vomiting is forceful and often upsetting for your baby. If your baby is repeatedly vomiting or there is blood in the vomit, it is time to get them medically reviewed.
- **Difficulty breathing:** It is a good idea to record your baby's normal breathing when awake and asleep on your phone. Make sure you lift their vest up and video their chest movement. If you think your baby's breathing has changed, you can compare it to this recording. If you notice that your baby is breathing faster than normal or appears to have to work harder to breathe (belly breathing), you should get them seen by a doctor.
- **Change in skin colour:** A sudden change in skin colour – such as bluish, grey, or mottled discolouration – can be a sign of illness. On black or

brown skin this may be easier to see on the palms of the hands or the soles of the feet.
- ***Rash:*** If your newborn develops a new rash, you should get them reviewed by a doctor. You need to get urgent medical attention if you roll a glass over it and can still see the rash whilst pressing down on the glass (this is a 'non-blanching' rash).
- ***Seizures:*** If your newborn has a seizure or convulsion, call the emergency services immediately.
- ***You sense that something is seriously wrong:*** All parents are the experts in their own child, and if you have a serious concern about your child, bring them to your own GP or, if that is not possible, an out-of-hours GP service or the emergency department.

If it is safe to do so, taking a video recording of anything unusual you observe can be very useful as this can be shown to the doctor.

CONGRATULATIONS!

Your little bundle of joy is now six weeks old and beginning to take in the world around them. They will kick their little legs and seek out your voice and your face. There is nothing in the world more fascinating to them than you. And I am sure the feeling is mutual.

CHAPTER 3
7 to 12 Weeks

Weeks 7 to 12 are a period of rapid growth and development for your baby, and, by the end of this time, you and your baby will have completed what is often called the 'fourth trimester'. At 12 weeks, your baby will have changed from a helpless newborn to an engaged and interactive little one. If you are first-time parents, you might also be feeling that newborn fog lifting, as sleep patterns change and you get longer stretches of sleep yourself, helping you to feel more refreshed.

FEEDING

Your baby's rate of weight gain might slow down after week six. Your baby will gain about 100–150 grams per week, and the average weight for a 12-week-old baby is 6 kilograms (13 pounds). Breastfed babies tend to gain weight more rapidly than formula-fed babies in the first 12 weeks.

If you are breastfeeding, your supply will usually be established by week seven, and you and your baby will have a good feeding routine going. By now most breastfed babies have a good latch and suck but, if any issues are persisting, it is important to speak to your GP, public-health nurse or lactation consultant. As long as your baby is gaining weight at a good rate and seems full and satisfied after a feed, you can be quite confident that they are getting enough milk. Growth spurts are common in breastfed babies, so they may go through phases of wanting to feed non-stop and then appear to grow overnight! This can be really tiring if you are doing the breastfeeding, so make sure to look after yourself during these growth spurts.

Formula-fed babies continue to need 150 millilitres of formula per kilogram of body weight over 24 hours. So, a 5-kilogram baby will need 750 millilitres over 24 hours, divided into six to eight feeds. Your baby might take bigger volumes of milk less frequently as they grow, so they might change from eight 95-millilitre feeds to six 125-millilitre feeds. You can start to figure out if your baby is ready to space out their feeds by offering them bigger volumes with each bottle, and then measuring how much is left over after each feed. You should continue to be led by your baby's hunger cues rather than trying to introduce a strict feeding schedule.

Feeding problems and faltering growth

By now most babies are on track with growth, but some babies may fall behind or stall in their weight gain. Some babies may be experiencing symptoms of reflux, cow's-milk-protein intolerance (CMPI), or, rarely, oral aversion.

Reflux might have been present from soon after birth or might only start to become obvious as your baby gets a little older. It is very common for babies under three months to spit up after feeds, as the junction between the food pipe (oesophagus) and the stomach is still developing. However, if your baby is showing the following signs (at any time in their first year), they may be experiencing reflux:

- coughing or hiccupping during feeding
- being unsettled during or after feeding
- refusing feeds or only taking small amounts

- gagging or choking during feeding because of regurgitating milk
- poor weight gain
- arching of the back.

Babies don't have to be spitting up milk to experience symptoms of reflux. If you notice any of the symptoms listed, speak to your GP or public-health nurse. The usual treatment offered by your GP will be either a thickener to add to the baby's formula or a special thickened formula. If your baby is breastfed, the thickener can be given to your baby before a feed. They may prescribe a proton pump inhibitor (such as omeprazole) to reduce the acidity in the stomach, which makes the reflux less uncomfortable. For formula-fed babies, they may recommend a change of formula.

Formula-fed babies with cow's-milk-protein allergy (CMPA) are usually diagnosed soon after birth, as they may have symptoms of rash, vomiting and diarrhoea soon after drinking a cow's-milk-based formula. However, cow's-milk-protein intolerance (CMPI) may only become obvious as your baby gets older.

If your baby is irritable and gassy after feeds, if they are passing lots of mucousy stools, or if they have blood in their stools, they may have CMPI. Your GP will likely advise you to first switch to an extensively hydrolysed (broken-down) formula. And if that doesn't help after two weeks, they might advise you to switch to an amino-acid-based formula, in which the proteins in the milk are broken down into their amino-acid building blocks. This means there is no cow's-milk protein left for your baby to react to. These specialised formulas taste quite different to cow's-milk formula, so it may take a while for your baby to get used to them.

Oral aversion is a sensitivity or fear of anything entering the mouth, and it can start to manifest itself in very young babies. It is a rare problem, which is more likely to occur in babies who were born prematurely or who had a stay and procedures in the neonatal-intensive-care unit (NICU) for other reasons. Most babies who are graduates of the NICU are linked in with multidisciplinary teams on discharge. If your baby was in NICU and you notice them turning away from the breast or bottle when it is offered, displaying a strong dislike of anything touching their mouth, or having a very sensitive gag reflex, then make sure to raise your concerns with your paediatrician. If your baby was never in NICU but is displaying these signs, discuss it with your GP or public-health nurse. Babies with reflux sometimes develop oral-aversion symptoms because they associate feeds with discomfort. However, this is quite rare.

Babies who have ongoing feeding difficulties or faltering growth between weeks 7 and 12, despite formula changes and treatment of possible reflux, are likely to need onward referral to a paediatrician for investigations and treatment.

POOP

By week seven, most babies have settled into a fairly regular pattern of passing bowel motions. Formula-fed babies will have between two and four dirty nappies a day, with the stool a toothpaste consistency. If you notice the stools becoming more pebble-like, if your baby is straining to pass a stool, or if they have not passed a stool for three or more days, you should speak to your GP as there is a possibility your baby is constipated. Blood in the stool or very pale, almost white stools are another indication you should speak to your GP. Do not offer your baby cooled boiled water in between feeds to relieve constipation unless advised to do so by a GP or nurse.

Breastfed babies can have very different patterns of passing stools. Some babies will have a dirty nappy after every feed, whereas others may go several days without passing a stool at all. If your breastfed baby has a sudden change in bowel habit, such as going from very frequent dirty nappies to very infrequent, hard stools, they may be constipated. Similarly, if they have a sudden change from infrequent stools to multiple dirty nappies a day, they may have an upset tummy. Sudden changes in bowel habits, blood in the stools, or very pale stools in breastfed babies warrant discussion with your GP.

PEE

Your 7-to-12-week-old baby will have about six to eight wet nappies a day. Once a week, it is good to make a note of how many wet nappies they have per day so that you can be alerted early to signs of dehydration if your baby is sick and not drinking as well as usual. Having fewer than half the usual number of wet nappies in a day is an early sign of dehydration, and having only one or two wet nappies in 24 hours is a clear sign of dehydration. If you notice decreased wet nappies in your baby, seek medical attention.

Urinary tract infections (UTIs) in babies under three months can be extremely serious, even life-threatening. There can be some subtle clues, such as upset or discomfort while peeing, or an unusual smell from the urine. However, the most common signs of a UTI will be vomiting, fever, and irritability. Fever (38°C or higher) can be a late sign, so if your baby develops new vomiting that is forceful (as opposed to posseting or reflux), you will need to get them checked by a doctor. Fever in any baby under three months old needs medical review, and the urine must always be checked for infection.

DEVELOPMENTAL MILESTONES

Your baby will continue to reach new milestones over the next six weeks. Your public-health nurse usually offers a 12-week developmental check, and it is important to attend.

Gross motor skills

Your baby's head and trunk control will continue to get stronger, so that, by 12 weeks old, they should be able to lift their head up without too much difficulty when you lay them on their tummy. They might be able to hold their head up and look around for a minute or two. By 12 weeks, some babies will begin to attempt rolling. If you notice this, you need to stop the use of swaddles and also be extra careful when placing your baby on a raised surface, such as a changing table, bed, or sofa.

Fine motor skills

Your baby's fine motor skills and vision will also be progressing. In the early days, you might have noticed that your baby often squinted when trying to focus their eyes but, by 12 weeks, squinting should no longer be evident.

Between 7 and 12 weeks, your baby will discover their hands. They might spend long periods of time staring at their hands; then, by 12 weeks, they might bring their hands together in front of their face and into their mouth. They will also start reaching out for objects and batting at them with open hands. In these six weeks, your baby will start to get enjoyment from a simple baby gym with brightly coloured objects that they can reach for and kick.

Communication and hearing

Your baby's hearing is becoming more acute, and they will turn their head to the source of a sound or a voice. They will also become increasingly vocal, with lots of cooing.

Social and emotional milestones

Your baby is becoming increasingly social as well with responsive smiling. Some babies may even have started to laugh by 12 weeks of age.

SLEEP

Babies still need a significant amount of sleep between the ages of 7 and 12 weeks – on average, they need 14–17 hours of sleep per 24 hours.

As the weeks go by, you will start to notice that they are learning the difference between night and day, and that the majority of their sleeping takes place at night. The times your baby will need to nap can vary from day to day, so make sure you continue to watch for sleep cues, such as yawning, eye-rubbing, or fussiness.

This is a good age to introduce a sleep routine in the evenings. For my babies, it was a short bath followed by some gentle baby massage, into a sleep onesie and their sleep sack, followed by a song or a story in dimmed light whilst being fed, and then being gently placed in their cot. These moments gave my babies the signal that it was bedtime and were precious at the end of each day. You will find a routine that works for you. The important thing is that you are consistent with it.

VACCINES

Vaccines are a crucial step in protecting your baby from serious and potentially life-threatening diseases. The first vaccines for your baby are offered at eight weeks. This is eight weeks 'chronological age', so even if your baby was born prematurely, it is their age on the calendar that matters when it comes to vaccines.

Why begin the vaccination schedule at eight weeks? This is

something that has been carefully studied to ensure that babies get the optimum benefit.

Newborns inherit some immunity from their mothers, particularly through antibodies transferred during pregnancy. This is called 'passive immunity'. However, this passive immunity diminishes rapidly in the first few weeks of life, leaving babies vulnerable to serious infections. Administering vaccines at eight weeks helps build the baby's immune response before exposure to these illnesses occurs. The timing is designed to provide protection during the critical early months when babies are most at risk of severe complications from these diseases.

Most vaccines will be administered in your baby's thigh, apart from the rotavirus vaccine, which is given orally. Some babies cry a little, but giving them something to suck on, such as a soother, or feeding them, can help to relieve any pain and quickly soothes them.

Vaccines administered at eight weeks

At eight weeks, your baby will receive the following vaccines:

- 6-in-1 vaccine
- PCV (Pneumococcal conjugate vaccine)
- Rotavirus oral vaccine.

The 6-in-1 vaccine targets the following six diseases:

- Diphtheria: Diphtheria is a bacterial infection that affects the nose, throat, and sometimes skin. It can cause breathing problems, heart failure, and even death. Vaccination has drastically reduced cases worldwide.
- Tetanus: Tetanus, sometimes called 'lockjaw', is a serious bacterial infection that affects the nervous system and causes muscle stiffness. It can lead to extreme difficulty with breathing and may cause death. The bacteria live in soil and can enter the body through cuts or wounds.

- Pertussis (whooping cough): Pertussis is a highly contagious bacterial infection that causes severe coughing fits. In babies, it can lead to serious complications such as pneumonia, seizures, and brain damage. It can also lead to death in small babies due to abnormal pauses in breathing (apnoea).
- Polio: Polio is a viral infection that can cause paralysis and even death. While rare in many parts of the world, vaccination is essential to ensure it remains under control.
- Haemophilus influenzae type b (Hib): Hib is a bacterial infection that can lead to severe illnesses, such as meningitis, pneumonia, and bloodstream infections, which are particularly dangerous for young children.
- Hepatitis B: Hepatitis B is a viral infection that affects the liver and can become chronic.

The other two vaccines given to your child at eight weeks protect them against the following:

- Pneumococcal disease: Pneumococcal bacteria can cause serious illnesses, such as pneumonia, meningitis, and blood infections. The PCV vaccine helps protect against these potentially life-threatening conditions.
- Rotavirus: Rotavirus is a highly contagious virus that causes severe diarrhoea, vomiting, and fever in young children. The oral vaccine is highly effective in preventing rotavirus infection.

Vaccine hesitancy

It is natural to have concerns about vaccines. However, scientific research consistently shows that they are safe and effective. They are rigorously tested before approval and continuously monitored for safety.

Concerns about vaccine safety grew in the late 1990s after a now-discredited study falsely linked the MMR vaccine (given at 12 months of age) to autism. That study, led by Andrew Wakefield, was later retracted because of ethical violations and flawed data. Wakefield was struck off the UK medical register due to findings of serious professional misconduct. Wakefield was found to have failed to obtain the correct ethical approval for his study, subjected children to painful and unnecessary procedures, and failed to disclose conflicts of interest and financial interests. Several large studies since the publication of Wakefield's paper have shown no link between MMR and autism.

Still, the effects of that misinformation linger, often amplified on social media. Some parents may feel overwhelmed or distrustful. This is understandable, and asking questions does not make you anti-vaccine, it makes you a caring, thoughtful parent.

The difference between misinformation (false but shared in error) and disinformation (deliberately misleading) is important. Seek trusted sources such as:

- In Ireland, HSE (hse.ie)
- In the UK, NHS (nhs.uk)
- World Health Organization (who.int)
- GP or public-health nurse.

Healthcare professionals are there to support you, not judge you.

Vaccination is a personal choice but one with public-health consequences. These vaccines protect not just your child, but other vulnerable people in the community who cannot be vaccinated for medical reasons.

Your baby's reaction to a vaccine will, generally, be mild and temporary. The diseases they prevent are often severe and, in some cases, fatal. Choosing to vaccinate your child is a step towards protecting them during their early years.

If you have concerns or questions, reach out. Honest, open

conversations with healthcare professionals can make a world of difference. Your child's well-being is at the heart of these decisions.

Common vaccine side-effects

After vaccination, some babies may experience mild side-effects, such as:

- redness or swelling at the injection site
- mild fever (remember, if your baby has a fever at less than three months of age, they should be medically reviewed)
- irritability or tiredness
- temporary loss of appetite.

These side-effects are usually mild and resolve within a day or two. Serious side-effects, such as allergic reaction, are extremely rare.

HEAD SHAPE

You might notice that the back of your baby's head looks flattened or lopsided. The medical term for a flattened head is 'brachycephaly' and the term for a lopsided head is 'plagiocephaly'. These head shapes are common and are usually due to positioning. A flattened head can occur if your baby prefers lying on their back, and a lopsided head shape can occur if your baby prefers looking to one side over the other.

If you notice an unusual head shape developing in your baby, speak to your GP or public-health nurse. For a flattened head shape, the treatment is usually increasing tummy time when your baby is awake. For a lopsided head shape, the management is usually physiotherapy to loosen out neck tightness, changing your baby's position in the cot so they need to turn the other way to look out, and placing interesting toys on their less preferred side when they are on their play mat. Specialised helmets are available in some countries to help mould the baby's head into a more symmetrical shape, but these helmets are not widely available in Ireland or the UK.

In rare cases, an abnormal head shape can be due to premature closure of one or more of the sutures in your baby's skull and, if this is the case, your baby will need specialised investigations and treatment.

ILLNESS

Despite your best efforts, your baby may well develop their first viral illness before they reach 12 weeks of age. This is especially true if they have older siblings who might be bringing home viruses from daycare or school. There are some things you can do to lower the risk of your little baby catching a viral infection, such as getting older siblings to change their clothes and wash their hands on arriving home, ensuring that visiting friends and relatives do not have any obvious signs of illness, and keeping your circle of contacts small – but, even doing all of this, your baby may become exposed to viral illness, so don't feel too bad if your baby develops a sniffle.

If they have symptoms of a cold, they may feel uncomfortable and find it difficult to feed. This is because babies breathe primarily through their nose, so a blocked nose makes it very hard to co-ordinate swallowing and breathing! You can try placing a few drops of normal saline (available in pharmacies) in your baby's nose, followed by gentle suction with a suction bulb. There are commercial suction devices available that are battery-run or hook up to a vacuum cleaner, but overly aggressive or frequent suctioning can actually make nasal secretions worse.

Your baby may also have a sore ear or a sore throat but, of

course, they can't tell you this, so if you suspect your baby is in pain after they are eight weeks old, you can give them a small dose of infant paracetamol (such as Calpol) as instructed by your pharmacist or GP. **Remember, if your baby has a fever of 38°C or more under the age of 12 weeks, they must be reviewed by a doctor.**

Your baby may also be drinking less than usual, so keep an eye on the number of wet nappies they are having and seek medical attention if it's fewer than half their usual number.

BRIEF RESOLVED UNEXPLAINED EVENT (BRUE)

One of the most frightening things that can happen is when a baby goes suddenly limp, pale, seems to choke, or goes blue around the lips. This can happen to babies up to the age of one, and if it is short-lived, and your baby responds to some stimulation or patting on the back, it will most likely be labelled a Brief Resolved Unexplained Event (BRUE). Usually, by the time the baby is receiving medical care, they are completely back to normal. You, on the other hand, will probably feel pretty shook.

So what is a BRUE, and why do they happen? The answer is, we don't really know why some babies have a BRUE. It may be that they choke on a little bit of vomit. It may be that they have a longer than normal pause in their breathing. They may have an underlying infection. In babies who are otherwise healthy, a cause is seldom found, although if your baby does have a BRUE they will be carefully observed and examined to rule out any underlying medical condition. However, most BRUEs are not a sign of any underlying medical problem, and in most babies, there is a low risk of it happening again, or leading to anything serious.

> If something like this does happen to your baby, make sure you care for yourself after the episode. Speak to family and loved ones, and get support from your GP or public-health nurse if you think you might need it.

The red flags for illness in this age group are the same as for babies aged two to six weeks. If you notice these signs in your baby, you need to seek immediate medical attention:

- **Fever:** A temperature of 38°C or above if they are under three months old.
- **Excessive fussiness:** Your baby may be impossible to console and their cry may have a different tone to usual. For example, it may sound high-pitched.
- **Bulging fontanelle:** The soft spot at the top of your baby's head is usually level with the rest of their scalp. If the skin over the soft spot starts to bulge upwards, it can be a sign of raised pressure around the brain, so your baby will need to be medically assessed.
- **Signs of dehydration:** When your baby is dehydrated, either due to reduced fluid intake or increased loss through vomiting or diarrhoea, they may have a reduced number of wet nappies, reduced tear production, and a sunken fontanelle.
- **Excessive sleepiness:** Your baby may be sleeping more than normal or not waking for feeds as normal. Excessive sleepiness may mean decreased consciousness, which is a sign of serious illness.

- **Vomiting:** You will be used to your baby spitting up small amounts of milk after feeds. This posseting is normal and effortless, while vomiting is forceful and often upsetting for your baby. If your baby is repeatedly vomiting or there is blood in the vomit, it is time to get them medically reviewed.
- **Difficulty breathing:** It is a good idea to record your baby's normal breathing when they are awake and asleep on your phone. Make sure you lift their vest up and video their chest movement. If you think your baby's breathing has changed, you can compare it to this recording. If you notice that your baby is breathing faster than normal or appears to have to work harder to breathe (belly breathing), you should get them seen by a doctor.
- **Change in skin colour:** A sudden change in skin colour, such as bluish, grey or mottled discolouration, can be a sign of illness. On black or brown skin this may be easier to see on the palms of the hands or the soles of the feet.
- **Rash:** If your newborn develops a new rash, you should get them reviewed by a doctor. You need to get urgent medical attention if you roll a glass over the rash and can still see it whilst pressing down on the glass (this is a 'non-blanching' rash).
- Seizures: If your newborn has a seizure or convulsion, call the emergency services immediately.
- **If you sense that something is seriously wrong:** All parents are the experts in their own child and if you have a serious concern about your child, bring them to your own GP or, if that is not possible, out-of-hours GP services or the emergency department.

CONGRATULATIONS!

Well done, your baby has officially completed their 'fourth trimester'. You can look forward to lots of fun and play and laughter in the weeks and months to come.

If this is your first baby, you have also made the transition into parenthood. By week 12, you will probably be feeling more confident in your parenting and getting longer stretches of sleep. Hopefully your own physical and mental health are good. Please remember to keep checking in with yourself – if you ever feel that low mood, anxiety, or exhaustion are threatening to overwhelm you, make sure to speak to your GP about your own health.

CHAPTER 4
4 to 6 Months

Your baby is now turning four months old, and lots more growth and development lie ahead. In the coming months, your baby will learn how to roll, how to control their hands, and how to utterly charm everyone who meets them!

FEEDING

By four months of age, your baby will probably have doubled their birth weight. So, a 3-kilogram baby might weigh 6 kilograms by month four. The amount of food they require is largely unchanged compared with the first three months. A breastfed baby might feed for longer, and your supply may change. Typically, they will look for about six feeds a day. Formula-fed babies continue to need 150 millilitres per kilogram, so a 6-kilogram baby will need 900 millilitres of formula milk, divided into approximately six feeds – so that's 150 millilitres per feed. Babies do not gain weight as rapidly as they did when aged under four months and, on average, you can expect your baby to gain about 20 grams per day, or 120–140 grams per week.

Between four and six months, your baby may start to show interest in solid food. Signs they may be ready to start weaning include:

- being able to sit while supported with good head control
- an increased interest in what you are eating
- co-ordination, including the ability to pick up objects and place them in their mouth.

It is not recommended to start weaning your baby before 17 weeks of age. If your baby was premature, use their corrected age (chronological age minus the number of weeks they were born early, e.g. minus 12 weeks for a baby born at 28 weeks) when making decisions about weaning. Risks associated with weaning before 17 weeks include tummy upset and suppression of appetite. Furthermore, your baby's kidneys are not mature enough to handle anything other than breast or formula milk until 17 weeks of age.

You should start your baby on solid foods by six months of age, because there are also downsides to delaying weaning beyond this, including iron deficiency. As your baby's iron stores are depleted by six months, they need more energy than can be provided by breast milk or formula alone. Also, the skills involved in chewing and swallowing are important for the development of speech. (See page 104 for more on weaning.)

Food allergies

Many parents fear the development of allergies when they start weaning their baby. However, it is important not to avoid allergens in babies with no underlying risk factors for food allergies, as delaying the introduction of allergenic foods can actually contribute to the development of allergy to those foods.

Dairy, peanut, and egg should be introduced at the same time as other solid food (for safety, nuts should be introduced in the form of smooth nut butter). Other allergens to introduce include fish, sesame seeds, tree nuts (almond, Brazil, cashew, hazelnut, walnut) and wheat.

Nevertheless, if your child does develop allergies, it is important that you don't listen to any 'well-meaning' friends or relatives who imply that your baby's allergies are somehow your fault. This comes from people having little information, a poor understanding of the complexities of food allergies, and a severe lack of tact! It is *not* your fault if your baby or child develops any allergies.

IgE-mediated allergies

There is a chance that your baby may have an allergic reaction when you start weaning them. However, this risk is small, and the risk of a more dangerous type of allergic reaction, called 'anaphylaxis', is even smaller.

Allergic reactions that have a rapid onset (within two hours) are due to IgE-mediated allergies. The body has antibodies, called IgE antibodies, towards certain foods. When that allergenic food is ingested, the antibodies activate, triggering certain cells in the body to release histamines that, in turn, lead to the symptoms of an allergic reaction.

Here are some signs that your baby may be allergic to a food you have introduced:

- an itchy or runny nose and/or sneezing
- a rash around the mouth
- hives and itchy skin
- tummy pain or a single episode of vomiting.

If you notice some of these symptoms, make note of what your child has eaten and stop feeding them the food you think they are reacting to. If safe to do so, take photographs of any rash and speak to your doctor. If your child is displaying several symptoms at once, call emergency services (999/112).

Anaphylaxis is a life-threatening emergency. The risk of anaphylaxis is extremely small in a weaning baby, but it is worth knowing what to look out for because the consequences of untreated anaphylaxis are so serious.

Here are some signs that your baby may be having an anaphylactic reaction to an allergen:

- breathlessness, wheezing, or repetitive coughing
- pale or bluish skin. On black or brown skin this may be easier to see on the palms of the hands or the soles of the feet
- swelling of the face, lips, or tongue
- widespread hives on the body
- repeated vomiting or diarrhoea
- suddenly being very tired, lethargic, or limp.

If your baby shows any of these symptoms, stop feeding them, call the emergency services immediately, and make it clear you think your baby is having an anaphylactic reaction. The first-line treatment of anaphylaxis is an adrenaline injection, and this information will help the paramedics to arrive prepared.

Non-IgE-mediated allergies

More rarely, babies may have a non-IgE-mediated reaction to a food. These types of allergic reaction are less well understood than IgE-mediated ones. They have a delayed onset, sometimes arising 24 hours or more after exposure to certain foods. The symptoms are mainly tummy based, and include tummy bloating, vomiting, and diarrhoea.

Types of non-IgE-mediated allergies include:

- Food protein-induced enterocolitis syndrome (FPIES): Characterised by severe vomiting, diarrhoea, and, sometimes, shock, often triggered by cow's milk or soy protein.

- Food protein-induced allergic proctocolitis (FPIAP): Affects the rectum, causing blood-streaked and mucousy stools in infants.
- Cow's-milk-protein intolerance (CMPI): A common type of non-IgE-mediated allergy, especially in infants (this can arise in breastfed babies who are exposed to dairy for the first time).

PEE AND POOP

I have grouped pee and poop together in this chapter because you should be into a predictable routine with your baby's nappies by month four.

The number of wet nappies your baby has each day is a good indicator of how well hydrated they are, so, every few weeks, track the number of wet nappies per day so that you know what their baseline is. A sudden drop in the number of wet nappies could be a sign of dehydration.

Babies between four and six months might experience constipation. Parents may be told by friends and family to give the baby cooled boiled water, but it is not advised to give babies water until they are over six months old. You should only give your baby water if advised to do so by a healthcare professional.

Constipation can be a little more common as you are weaning your baby, as their system gets used to solid food.

As we discussed in Chapter 2, constipation can be managed in the following ways:

- a warm bath and gentle tummy massage to help your baby's bowels to move
- 'bicycling' your baby's legs by gently moving them up and down while they are lying on their back.

Your baby should be seen by a doctor for their constipation if they have any of these symptoms:

- it lasts more than two days
- they are very distressed
- you feel very concerned
- they have a fever
- their appetite decreases
- they start to vomit
- their tummy is bloated or distended
- they develop bloody stools
- they stop gaining or start losing weight.

SKIN

At this age, your baby's skin is delicate and can be sensitive. Use soft fabrics for your baby's base layer of clothing (i.e. vests) and use fragrance-free, 'non-bio' detergents when doing laundry. This is because 'biological', or 'bio', detergents contain enzymes that break down dirt, but that can also irritate a baby's skin.

Any soap or moisturiser you use on your baby should be fragrance-free and designed for babies. After a bath, make sure your baby's skin is fully dry, especially in those lovely creases under their neck and in their armpits.

Between four and six months, your baby might start to dribble or drool more. This saliva, which may contain milk or spit-up or food, can irritate the skin around the mouth, on the chin, and under the chin. Rather than rubbing the drool, make sure you dab it away. Putting a thin layer of petroleum jelly (Vaseline) on and under the chin can also form a barrier and protect the skin.

Nappy rash

Most babies will have at least one bout of nappy rash and, having been there as a parent, I know that feeling a bit guilty about this is common. But nappy rash is part and parcel of babyhood, and there is no need to feel guilty. It is usually easy to treat and, when you know how to spot the early signs and identify the triggers, prevention can be pretty straightforward too.

Nappy rash typically appears as red, sore patches on the skin around the nappy area – usually the bottom, thighs, or genitals. The skin may look inflamed, feel warm to the touch, or appear shiny. Your baby might seem uncomfortable during nappy changes or when the area is cleaned.

Nappy rash can be triggered by a variety of things, including:

- Prolonged contact with pee or poo: This is the most common cause – when a nappy isn't changed quickly enough, moisture and waste irritate the skin.
- Chafing or rubbing: Tight nappies or rough materials can cause friction on your baby's sensitive skin.
- New products: Sometimes wipes, detergents, or bubble baths can cause a reaction, especially if they contain fragrances or alcohol.
- Antibiotics: Whether your baby is taking them or you're on them while breastfeeding, antibiotics can upset the balance of bacteria on your baby's skin, increasing the risk of a rash or yeast infection.

Nappy rash can usually be treated at home. Change nappies frequently, leave nappies off for periods during the day to let that little bottom dry off fully, clean the area using a cloth or cotton wool and warm water, and apply a preparation of zinc oxide that is suitable for babies (your pharmacist will give you good advice).

Sometimes, your baby's nappy rash might need medical attention, and your doctor may prescribe a medicated cream if there's an infection present.

You should speak to a doctor if:

- the rash doesn't improve within three days of home treatment
- the skin is broken, blistered, or oozing
- your baby seems very uncomfortable or develops a fever
- the rash spreads beyond the nappy area
- you suspect a yeast or bacterial infection.

Here are some easy steps to reduce the chances of nappy rash recurring:

- Change nappies regularly, even overnight.
- Clean the area gently but thoroughly at each change.
- Use a barrier cream daily (e.g. petroleum jelly) to protect the skin.
- Give your baby some nappy-free time every day to let their skin breathe.
- Choose nappies that fit well and enable airflow; avoid tight clothes that cause friction.
- Be cautious with new products, and test them on a small area of skin before full use.

Eczema

Eczema can affect up to 20% of babies under the age of two – that's one in every five babies! The good news is that lots of babies outgrow their eczema, but it is important to manage the condition carefully to help keep your baby comfortable, because eczema is itchy!

In babies under six months, eczema typically appears on the

cheeks, forehead, and scalp, although it can also appear on the arms, legs, or torso. The skin may look red, rough, and scaly, or it may even be oozing in more severe cases.

If you notice a new rash on your baby, it is important first to get them reviewed by their GP. If they are diagnosed with eczema, you will be given information on how to manage it. Don't forget that your pharmacist will also be able to give you lots of information about good products to use.

The most important part of eczema treatment is keeping the skin moisturised. Use moisturising products that are designed for babies and are fragrance-free. The skin will be itchy and even tiny baby fingernails can do damage when scratching, so keep fingernails short and consider mittens to cover the hands when your baby is asleep to prevent scratching.

Check your baby's skin daily for signs of a worsening rash or infection. Try to monitor what causes your baby's eczema to flare up. Certain fabrics, skin products, washing detergents, or soaps might irritate your baby's skin, so remove these triggers if possible. The fabric closest to your baby's skin should be natural, light, and breathable, such as cotton.

If your baby's eczema is worse despite all these precautions, you should get them checked by your GP, who may prescribe a topical steroid to be used for a short period of time.

Eczema and allergies

Babies with eczema are also statistically more likely to develop food allergies. However, not all babies with eczema develop food allergies. It is important to wean your baby in the usual way, and not to delay the introduction of allergens, such as dairy, egg, and nuts, unless advised to by your baby's doctor.

Babies and children with eczema are also more prone to developing asthma and hay fever when they are older. Remember, if this happens, it is largely due to genetics; there is nothing you have done wrong as a parent.

Cradle cap

Cradle cap is a harmless skin condition caused by the build-up of dry skin and natural oils on your baby's scalp. Its medical term is 'seborrheic dermatitis'. The main symptoms are patches of greasy, scaly skin, mainly on the scalp, but it can be present on the eyebrows and even in the nappy area. The skin is not itchy and cradle cap does not cause your baby any discomfort.

Tempting as it may be, it is important not to pick at the scales to try and remove them. Instead, apply moisturiser or baby oil to the area. Do not use food-based oils like olive oil or peanut oil. After applying moisturiser or oil, gently brush or massage your baby's scalp, then wash with baby shampoo. Your pharmacist will give you good advice on the best moisturisers, oils, and shampoos to use. Don't be too alarmed if little patches of hair come away with the cradle cap scales. This is common, and the hair will grow back.

DEVELOPMENTAL MILESTONES

When they turn four months old, your baby is lying on their back, gazing at their hands, and trying to figure them out, and, at six months, they are rolling, maybe trying to sit up, and grabbing everything within reach. So much happens with your baby's development in what feels like the blink of an eye.

By now, you might be getting out and about and meeting other parents and babies, and you may end up comparing your baby's milestones to other babies of the same age. If this is your second or third baby, you might even find yourself comparing them to their older siblings. One of my babies had lots of words by the age of one, but didn't walk until 14 months; whereas the other was walking at nine months! Remember, every baby develops at their own unique rate, and milestones are used by healthcare professionals to simply identify and manage any potential problems at an early stage.

Gross motor skills

The gross-motor milestone we expect babies aged six months to have reached is rolling. In order to be able to roll, a baby has to have mastered head and neck control and the ability to push themselves up on their arms, so a lot needs to happen before your baby does their first little roll. Usually, babies will start trying to roll between four and five months, but it might take some time for them to succeed! When they start rolling, they can roll *off* things, such as sofas, changing tables, and beds, so never leave your baby unattended on anything that is raised off the ground.

Some babies may be able to sit with support by six months, but don't worry too much if your baby is not doing this by this stage.

Fine motor skills

You'll notice a real progression in your baby's fine-motor control between three and six months. They will go from batting at objects with a pretty poor aim to being able to reach for something, pick it up, and transfer it from one hand to the other. If they drink from a bottle, they will be able to hold the bottle themselves for short periods, but you do need to continue to supervise your baby's bottle feeds. By six months, they can also place food and objects in their mouth, so be careful not to leave anything within reach that you don't want in your baby's mouth.

Fine motor skills and vision are closely linked, so if your baby is showing any delays in fine-motor development, they may also need their vision checked. By six months, your baby should not be showing any preference for one hand over the other, so if you notice a hand preference, or if one or both hands are held in a tight fist most of the time, make sure you mention it to your baby's doctor.

Communication and hearing

Your baby's language will be starting to develop at this stage. They will learn to recognise their own name. They may look closely at your mouth when you speak, and they may begin to babble in syllables by six months. Their hearing is very acute by now, and they will quickly turn their head to try and identify the source of a sound.

Social and emotional milestones

Socially, your baby will become more interactive with people and more interested in the world around them. They will recognise familiar faces and voices. They will begin to express emotions, such as happiness and frustration. You will start to hear your baby laughing. They really enjoy a 'back and forth' with their caregivers, so you will find yourself having entire conversations in gobbledygook. Enjoy them – some of my best conversations with my babies were in gobbledygook!

SLEEP

Have you been asked yet if your baby is a 'good sleeper'? What an irritating question that can become! If you're the parent of a baby between four and six months old, you're probably tired – and you might be wondering what's normal and what's not.

At this age, many babies start to develop more regular sleep patterns, but sleeping 'through the night' doesn't necessarily mean 12 straight hours. In fact, in medical terms, sleeping through the night often means a stretch of five to six hours, and that's not guaranteed every night.

Normal sleep at this stage includes:

- 2–3 daytime naps, with wake windows of 1.5 to 2.5 hours
- night sleep that may include one or more wakes for feeding
- a total of about 12–16 hours of sleep across a 24-hour period.

Every baby is different. Some may start giving you longer stretches at night, others will still wake multiple times; both are completely normal.

Is it sleep regression or just ... a baby?

Many parents notice sleep suddenly gets worse around four months. This is often referred to as the 'four-month sleep regression', but, really, it's a developmental progression.

Around this time, your baby's sleep cycles mature. They move from newborn-style deep sleep into more adult-like patterns, with lighter stages of sleep and more frequent wake-ups. It's not a step backwards, it's a sign their brain is developing. But, yes, it's exhausting!

Sleep safety

Sleep safety is crucial. The guidelines from the HSE (Ireland) and The Lullaby Trust (UK) both support these key principles:

- Back to sleep: Always place your baby on their back to sleep.
- Clear sleep space: Keep the cot or Moses basket clear of toys, bumpers, pillows, and loose blankets.
- Smoke-free environment: This dramatically reduces the risk of sudden infant death syndrome (SIDS).
- Room-sharing: Keep your baby in your room (in a separate sleep space) for the first six months.
- Breastfeeding: If it's possible to breastfeed, it provides protective benefits for both baby and mother.

VACCINES

Your baby will have two more rounds of vaccines between the ages of four and six months. The vaccines at four months are almost identical to those given at eight weeks, described on page 73. The only difference is that, at four months, your baby will not get a dose of the PCV vaccine.

The vaccines at six months are the 6-in-1 vaccine and the PCV vaccine. These are described on pages 73–4. In order to be fully protected against the illnesses listed on the vaccine schedule, your baby needs to receive all the recommended doses of each vaccine.

As your baby gets a little older, they might be more aware of the fact that they are in an unfamiliar environment, and they might cry a little more loudly and slightly longer after their vaccines compared to when they were a tiny eight-week-old. Distraction, in the form of toys or offering a soother or a feed at the time of the vaccine, can really help.

Your baby might develop some redness or swelling at the site of the vaccine on the thigh, or they might have a fever in the 48 hours after their vaccine. You can use paracetamol or ibuprofen to ease any discomfort or fever.

ILLNESSES

By now, you will probably be getting out and about more with your baby, so they will likely be interacting more with non-family members. This means that, as well as meeting new people, they are likely to encounter new viruses and bacteria. Don't worry, this is a normal part of babyhood and, as they grow, their immune system will be better able to cope with whatever germs they encounter.

I found my baby's first viral head cold hard to handle, even though the paediatrician part of my brain knew she would be just fine. I wanted to take away her discomfort (and snots!) and explain to her that she would be feeling better soon. She was just so unhappy and uncomfortable, and I knew this was the first of many viral illnesses to come.

Viral illnesses

Most viral illnesses in babies cause symptoms of a cold, or what your doctor might call an 'upper respiratory tract infection' (URTI). It is normal for babies and children to have between 6 and 12 viral illnesses per year – so, yes, it can sometimes feel like they are always sick!

Symptoms of a viral illness include runny nose, watery eyes, cough, and poor feeding. Your baby may also have a fever. You have been conditioned to get your baby checked immediately for a fever under the age of three months, so it can feel a bit daunting to manage your older baby's fever at home without going to the doctor. Remember, if you feel in any way uneasy or concerned about your baby's health, it is best to contact your GP.

The red flags for viral illness in babies aged four to six months which require immediate medical attention are:

- a fever for more than three days, fever that does not come down with medication (paracetamol or ibuprofen), or a fever of 39°C or more
- if your baby seems to be using their tummy muscles to breathe, is breathing faster than normal, or finds it hard to take their bottle or breastfeed due to being breathless

- fewer than three wet nappies in 24 hours or no wet nappy for 12 hours
- a change in the fontanelle (soft spot) on their head, either more sunken or bulging
- extreme irritability
- drowsy and not waking for feeds
- refusing to take feeds
- a change in skin colour, so that skin that looks bluish or grey, or mottled skin (for black or brown skin, this is most obvious on the palms of the hands or soles of the feet)
- a rash that does not disappear when you press down on the skin with a clear glass.

If your baby has a runny nose, a mild cough, or a low-grade fever and is not displaying any of the red flags on the list, here are some tips for managing viral illness at home:

- Dress your baby in their normal clothes, there is no need to strip them down or wrap them up.
- Offer them the breast or bottle frequently.
- Give regular paracetamol or ibuprofen – check the correct dose with your GP or pharmacist.
- Ensure your baby gets plenty of rest as they will be more tired than usual; it is best to stay at home for a few days.

Common viral illnesses

Most viruses prefer the colder weather, and, in paediatrics, we refer to the months between September and April as 'viral season'. Another way to think of it is if there is an 'R' in the month, it's probably still viral season (in the northern hemisphere). It is extremely hard to avoid viral infections, which can spread through the air, from surfaces, or through direct contact.

Here are some of the viruses your baby is most likely to encounter in the first year.

Rhinovirus

Rhinovirus is a large family with about 165 subtypes, and it is the main cause of the common cold ('rhino' means 'nose', so 'nose virus'). There is no vaccine for rhinovirus because of the large number of subtypes, and there is no specific treatment. It will take your baby between 4 and 10 days to recover from this virus and, initially, they may seem to get a little worse before they get better. However, if, after three to four days, they continue to get worse instead of beginning to improve, they should be reviewed by their GP or reviewed immediately if they show any of the red flags listed on pages 96–97.

Respiratory syncytial virus (RSV)

RSV is a very common virus that can affect people of any age, but it is more likely to cause bronchiolitis (a cough and wheeze) in children under the age of two, and it is more likely to cause serious illness needing hospitalisation in babies under six months.

RSV usually starts out like a cold, and your baby may have a mild fever, sneezing, and a runny nose. After a few days, your baby may start to get better but, in some babies, the infection then starts to cause symptoms in the chest, with a cough, rapid breathing, and increased use of muscles between the ribs and in the tummy when breathing. They may also develop a wheeze. The increased effort babies need to put into breathing means that sucking and feeding becomes more difficult. If you notice these symptoms in your baby, it is important to seek medical attention.

There is no specific treatment for RSV. If babies become unwell due to this virus and need to be hospitalised, they can be supported with their feeding and breathing as the virus runs its course. Supportive treatment measures include:

- Fluids: If your baby is unable to drink, they may get an IV (intravenous) line to give fluids and electrolytes.
- Oxygen: Extra oxygen can be given via a mask or nasal prong.
- Suctioning of mucus: To help clear your baby's nostrils and make it easier for them to breathe.
- Bronchodilator medicines: These may help to open your baby's airways.
- Tube feeding: This may be done if a baby has trouble sucking. They are fed via a thin tube that runs through the baby's nose and down into the stomach.
- Mechanical ventilation: Rarely, a baby who is very ill may need to be put on a breathing machine (ventilator) to help with their breathing.

All of this can be quite scary to read, but there are some measures you can take to prevent your baby catching RSV. The virus can be spread by droplets, surfaces, or direct contact. One of the most common ways a baby can catch RSV is via kisses and cuddles from someone who is infected, so it is important that older siblings and other relatives wash their hands before holding your baby and avoid kissing them on the face or hands.

Two major breakthroughs in the prevention of RSV have been:

- a vaccine that can be offered to pregnant mums between 32 and 36 weeks, allowing maternal antibodies to cross the placenta, giving the baby about six months' protection
- a monoclonal antibody medication called nirsevimab, which is usually offered soon after birth and given as an injection, that blocks the RSV from entering the baby's cells and provides about six months' protection.

Depending on which country you live in, one or the other of these options may be offered to you. Countries that are offering nirsevimab to babies in their first winter (this includes Ireland) are reporting an over 80% drop in babies needing to be hospitalised because of RSV.

Adenovirus

Adenovirus can cause similar symptoms to RSV, but, in addition to the breathing symptoms, such as cough and wheeze, your baby may have signs of red eyes (conjunctivitis) and tummy upset (vomiting and diarrhoea). Most cases of adenovirus are mild and resolve themselves, without specific medical treatment, but keep an eye out for the red flags listed on pages 96–97 and seek medical attention if you are concerned about your baby.

Hand, foot, and mouth disease

Hand, foot, and mouth disease is a very common and highly contagious viral illness that your baby (and also you) can catch more than once. It tends to affect babies under six months more severely than older babies and children, but in general it will resolve itself and will not need any specialised care.

The first symptom is usually a sore throat, so your baby may sound hoarse and not want to feed. They will also probably have a fever. You will then start to notice spots in and around the mouth, which look like little blisters. These spots will also appear on their hands and feet, and often appear in the nappy area as well.

Give your baby regular pain relief using paracetamol or ibuprofen (get your GP or pharmacist to check you are giving the correct dose for your baby's weight), and offer frequent drinks of breast milk or formula. If your baby is taking solids, offer bland, soft foods, such as rice or potatoes. Avoid citrus or anything spicy as this will cause the mouth blisters to sting.

Remember, viruses do not respond to antibiotics. The mainstays of treatment for viral illness are controlling pain and fever using paracetamol and ibuprofen, ensuring adequate hydration by offering frequent feeds, making sure your baby gets plenty of rest, and monitoring closely for the emergence of any red flags. If you notice any of the red flags from the list on pages 96–97, seek medical attention.

Bacterial illnesses

Bacterial infections are generally more serious than viral infections and will need medical attention and antibiotics. But how can you, as a parent or caregiver, tell the difference between something that is a simple virus and something that is potentially very serious? Well, the truth is, it is very unlikely that you will be able to tell the difference but, by being attuned to any possible red flags or signs of deterioration in your baby, you will be empowered to seek a medical review promptly and advocate for your baby's care.

Many bacterial infections in babies, children, and adults are known as 'secondary bacterial infections'. A secondary bacterial infection is basically one that uses an opportunity created by a viral infection in order to sneak past the immune system. Examples include tonsillitis or otitis media (ear infection) after a viral upper respiratory tract infection, or bacterial pneumonia after RSV bronchiolitis.

Younger babies are more susceptible to secondary bacterial infections because of their immature immune systems. Many parents and caregivers are told their baby has a 'viral' infection only for their baby to become more unwell and require antibiotics and possible hospitalisation. In most cases, the initial diagnosis of a viral illness was correct, but a secondary bacterial infection developed.

Here are some signs that your baby may be developing a bacterial infection:

- **Fever is a big indicator of bacterial infection.** Large population-based studies have shown that a fever (above 38°C) that persists for five days or more is significantly more likely to be caused by a bacterial infection than a viral infection. Any fever lasting five days or more warrants further investigation and possible referral to hospital for assessment.
- **Low temperature (below 36°C)** can also be a sign of a developing bacterial infection, so if your baby's temperature suddenly starts to drop, you should also seek medical attention.
- **An area of redness spreading on the body** that may feel hot to touch can be a sign of a bacterial skin infection.
- **A rash that does not fade when pressed with a clear glass** needs urgent assessment.
- **Irritability** may indicate a worsening of your baby's viral illness or the beginning of a bacterial infection.
- **Sleeping more than usual or not waking for feeds** can also be an indicator of infection.

As you can see, most of the signs of bacterial infection are indistinguishable from the red flags for all illnesses, so if you see any signs in your baby that are included in the list above or the one on pages 96–97, you can feel strongly empowered to advocate for your baby and get their care escalated if needed.

Urinary tract infection

Another cause of bacterial illness in babies is a urinary tract infection (UTI). UTIs can be very serious and need prompt medical attention in babies under six months. The early signs of a UTI can be very subtle:

- apparent pain or discomfort when peeing
- a different or strange smell from the urine
- very dark or reddish urine
- a change in the number of wet nappies
- vomiting
- fever
- rigors (looks like uncontrolled shivering).

You know your baby best. It can be very hard to see them unwell, but being familiar with which red flags to watch out for can empower you to act. Remember, if at any stage you have a gut feeling that something is not right, pay attention to that feeling and get your baby reviewed by a doctor.

CONGRATULATIONS!

So much happens in your baby's life between four and six months. It may feel like a whirlwind, but at the centre of all of it is your beautiful baby, and at the centre of your baby's universe is you.

Hopefully by now, you are feeling more rested and are settling into parenthood. Having your first baby is a big transition, but going from one to two or two to three is equally momentous in different ways. Just make sure, in the midst of all the glorious chaos, that you are taking care of yourself too.

CHAPTER 5
6 to 12 Months

Can you believe your baby is six months old? There are so many exciting things in store for your little one over the next six months and, at the end of it, you will celebrate their first birthday. Incredible!

FEEDING AND GROWTH

By six months, your baby may already have started weaning on to solids or may be just about ready to start. When your baby starts weaning, they will still get most of their nutrition from breast or formula milk but, by the time they are a year old, most of their calories will come from solid food.

It might be difficult to imagine this being the case as you start your baby's weaning journey. My first baby took to solid foods like a duck to water. With her very first mouthful of baby rice, her eyes opened wide with delight, as if to say, 'So long, milk, there's a new show in town!' My second baby was a lot more suspicious of the whole process, and she clearly preferred her mummy's milk to anything we offered her from a spoon. All babies are unique, and how they take to weaning is no exception.

Signs your baby might be ready to start weaning include:

- sitting up with little support
- good head and neck control
- showing interest in food (watching you eat, reaching out)
- losing the tongue-thrust reflex (so they don't push food out automatically).

Breast milk or formula should remain the main source of nutrition between 6 and 12 months, but as the amount of solid food your baby eats increases, the amount of breast or formula milk they need will decrease. Introducing solids adds new nutrients and experiences.

Follow-on formula

Follow-on formulas are marketed for babies from six months onwards, but they are not needed if your baby is eating a healthy, balanced diet. These formulas are fortified with extra iron and other nutrients, but most babies can get what they need from food after six months, along with continued breast milk or first formula up to 12 months.

First infant formula is the only type recommended for formula-fed babies in their first year, and there are no health benefits in switching to follow-on milk at any stage.

Safe mealtimes

When your baby is able to support themselves in a high chair, this is the safest place for them to eat, with an adult directly facing and supervising them. The high chair should have a five-point harness, which you *must* use. Many caregivers incorrectly believe that it is safer not to strap in the baby just in case they start to choke and need choking first aid. However, the risk of falling out of the high chair and being injured is far higher than the risk of choking, and it will only take seconds to undo the harness in the event that baby needs to be removed from the high chair quickly.

How much milk?

As your baby's intake of solid food increases, their intake of milk will decrease. At the start of weaning, offer your baby the usual amount of breast or bottle feeds. Offer milk *after* their solids.

If you are breastfeeding, you may notice your baby is looking for fewer feeds or spending less time on the breast. Bottle-fed babies may not finish their bottles or look for fewer bottles. Your baby will continue to have breast milk or formula milk as their main drink until age one, and will likely take four to six breast-feeds per day or 600 millilitres of formula.

First foods to try

Start simple! Single-ingredient, smooth-textured foods are best at first. Some popular first foods include:

- iron-fortified baby cereals (oat or rice cereal)
- puréed vegetables (sweet potato, carrot, peas)
- puréed fruits (apple, pear, banana)
- puréed meats (chicken, turkey, beef).

Offer small amounts (about a teaspoon at first) and gradually increase the amount as your baby shows interest. And wait three to five days between introducing new foods. This helps you identify any food allergies or sensitivities.

Moving to more textures

Around seven to nine months, your baby will likely be ready for:

- thicker purées
- mashed foods
- soft finger foods (cooked pasta, soft fruits, and scrambled egg).

This is also a good time to encourage self-feeding with safe, soft pieces of food your baby can grasp. It's messy, but it helps build motor skills and confidence.

Baby-led weaning and spoon-feeding

You may have heard about 'baby-led weaning', where the baby is encouraged to feed themselves without you feeding them by spoon. If your baby is only going to self-feed, then make sure that the food you offer is suitable for baby-led weaning, such as carrot and broccoli boiled until soft, or soft fruits, such as ripe mango cut into strips. If you can squash a food by gently pressing it between your index finger and thumb, your baby can usually chew it effectively.

Some parents prefer baby-led weaning and others prefer spoon-feeding, whilst many favour a mixture of both. There is no right or wrong way to wean your baby, as long as you and your baby are enjoying the process and your baby is getting to try lots of new and delicious tastes and textures.

Building a feeding routine

By about nine months of age, most babies benefit from three small meals a day, along with breast milk or formula feeds. Try to:

- offer meals at regular times
- let your baby eat with the family when possible
- encourage exploration and self-feeding.

Meals don't have to be elaborate – simple and nutritious is what you are aiming for! Here is a list of some important nutrients to incorporate during weaning:

- Iron: Crucial for brain development (meats, fortified cereals, lentils, beans)
- Zinc: Important for growth and immunity (meats, dairy, wholegrains)
- Healthy fats: Support brain and eye development (avocado, full-fat yogurt, oily fish).

It's important to ensure that food (especially eggs, meat and fish) is fully cooked. There are certain foods that should be avoided completely before the age of one. These are:

- honey (risk of botulism)
- whole nuts (choking hazard – use smooth nut butters instead)
- added salt and sugar
- unpasteurised cheeses or milk.

You can encourage a positive meal experience for both you and your baby by staying relaxed and patient. Let your baby touch, smell, and play with their food, and celebrate small successes, even if most of the meal ends up on the floor! It is important to respond to hunger and fullness cues – don't force your baby to finish their meal.

WHAT ABOUT GROWTH?

The first six months are characterised by rapid growth, and your six-month-old baby usually weighs at least double what they did as a newborn. In the next six months, your baby's rate of growth will slow down and they will gain, on average, 2 kilograms between the age of 6 and 12 months.

Your baby should be offered at least one review with the public-health nurse during this time, who will most likely plot your baby's length and weight on a centile chart. They will also measure your baby's head circumference and check it against the centile chart.

A centile chart, also known as a growth chart, is a visual tool used to track and assess a baby's growth and development. They show the average weight, length, and head circumference for babies of different ages, represented by curved lines, called 'centiles'. These charts help healthcare professionals monitor a baby's growth compared to other babies of the same age and sex.

Each baby is unique, but monitoring their growth helps healthcare professionals to check your baby's growth against population averages. It also helps to spot any change in your baby's own growth pattern; for example, if their weight falls down a percentile over a few months or their head size suddenly starts going up into the higher centiles.

By the age of one, the average baby boy weighs 10.3 kilograms and the average baby girl weighs 9.5 kilograms. The average head circumference goes from 34 centimetres at birth to 46 centimetres at age one.

PEE AND POOP

Your baby might start to produce less pee when they start eating solids, but they will still have six to eight wet nappies per day. Usually, baby's pee is clear or pale yellow. If it is much darker than usual, this may be a sign of dehydration. It's handy to make a note of how many wet nappies your baby usually has so that if they are sick or you notice a drop in the number of wet nappies, you will spot dehydration early.

The smell of pee changes sometimes after solids are started, but a strong or foul smell, or signs it hurts your baby to pee, might signal a urine infection. You should speak to your GP if you notice this.

Now that your baby is on solids, you can basically expect the rainbow when it comes to the colour of their poop. Poop can be yellow, brown, green, or even orange, depending on what your baby eats. Don't be alarmed by undigested food bits – that's common at this stage.

Stools will appear more formed and pastier compared to early baby poop. Some babies will have a bowel movement several times a day, while others may go only every couple of days. Both are normal, especially after solids are introduced. The key is that your baby seems comfortable and that the stools aren't hard or painful to pass.

DEVELOPMENTAL MILESTONES

All that head growth means your baby's brain is growing and developing quickly! And with that growth comes even more developmental milestones.

Remember that doctors and nurses ask about milestones so that they can identify any developmental issues early. We know that every baby is unique and develops at their own pace. Ignore anyone who tries to compare your baby with theirs – this is not a competition or a race!

Let's look at gross motor, fine motor, language, and social development from month to month. Your baby will be developing new skills rapidly!

Seven months
- Gross motor skills: By seven months, from a gross-motor perspective, your baby will be able to roll from front to back and back to front. They will most likely be able to sit with assistance, and some babies might be starting to scoot along the floor on their belly, although it won't look very graceful!
- Fine motor skills: Their fine-motor development will be coming along too, and they will be able to hold an object firmly in their hands by clutching it between their fingers and the palm of their hand, pass the object from one hand to another, and place it in their mouth.

- Language: Hearing is essential to speech-and-language development, and your baby should be able to turn their head to the source of a sound and recognise familiar voices. They will also probably know their own name by now. The babbling will really start to take off, and you'll have lots of entertaining interactions in 'baby language'.
- Social: Your baby will enjoy seeing new faces and new sights. They will show a clear preference for people they recognise, but they do not usually show stranger or separation anxiety at this age.

Eight months
- Gross motor skills: At eight months, your baby will be rolling, sitting, and maybe starting to crawl. They will probably be able to manoeuvre themselves from a lying to a sitting position.
- Fine motor skills: They will start to become more dexterous with their hands and start to show signs of a basic pincer grasp, which is holding small objects between their thumb and the side of their index finger.
- Language: More syllables will start to come through in their language, and they may repeat syllables. The first syllable is often 'da da da da' – the dads are usually delighted about this, the mums not so much!
- Social: By eight months, most babies really enjoy play, such as banging objects together, mimicking movements and facial expressions, and beginning to play peek-a-boo.

Nine months
- Gross motor skills: By nine months, many babies can crawl on their hands and knees, though some babies prefer to shuffle around on their bottom. Many nine-month-olds who can crawl or shuffle around will then try to use furniture, such as coffee tables or sofas, to pull themselves up into a standing position. When your baby can move around, it's

time to reassess your babyproofing measures and ensure all furniture is safely anchored so that your baby isn't able to pull it down on top of themselves.
- Fine motor skills: Your baby's fine motor skills will be going from strength to strength. They can grasp a cube or brick using their thumb and fingertips, as opposed to just clutching it in their palm, and their pincer grasp continues to improve.
- Language: Your baby's language also continues to develop. Nine-month-old babies are usually great communicators and are beginning to understand the non-verbal concepts of waving 'bye-bye' and pointing. The number of sounds they make increases, and 'mama' may even make an appearance! They don't use 'dada' specifically for their dad or 'mama' specifically for their mum, but this will come soon!
- Social: At around nine months, babies develop the concept of 'object permanence', meaning they understand that, even if an object is hidden, it is still there. For example, if they drop their spoon from the high chair, they will look for it – this then becomes a great game to see how many times you will pick it up for them! Nine-month-old babies also begin to develop wariness of people they don't recognise. This is called 'stranger anxiety'. They may also develop separation anxiety, which often manifests as tears and upset when being dropped off at daycare or with a childminder. This phase can be very tough for parents, who might feel guilty about having to leave their baby. I know I found it very difficult.

Ten months

- Gross motor skills: At 10 months, most babies are mobile, whether crawling or bottom-shuffling. They may also start 'cruising', i.e. taking sideways steps whilst holding on to furniture.

- Fine motor skills: From a fine motor skills point of view, most 10-month-olds discover their index finger, which they use to gently (or not so gently, in the case of your eye) poke at things.
- Language: Language continues to develop quickly, and your 10-month-old will begin to understand the word 'no' – and maybe even push some boundaries! They may begin to shake their own head to indicate 'no'. They will probably now have two words that have specific meanings: 'Dada' and 'Mama' – finally!
- Social: At 10 months, your baby will begin to appreciate applause, and they will understand the positive reinforcement you give them when you clap your hands and praise them.

Eleven months
- Gross motor skills: By 11 months, your baby may have mastered the art of cruising, and they may even stand unsupported for a few wobbly seconds.
- Fine motor skills: Their hand movements are becoming ever more refined, and they have begun to master that pincer grasp, so they can pick up and hold objects between their index finger and thumb.
- Language: As well as babbling, they may now start to copy sounds that you make, although they are unlikely to have any recognisable words apart from 'Dada' and 'Mama'.
- Social: By 11 months, your baby may start to develop a sense of self, for example recognising themselves in the mirror or in photos.

Twelve months
- Gross motor skills: At 12 months, your baby will have mastered the art of bottom-shuffling and pulling themselves up to stand. They may be expert cruisers and be able to stand alone for a little longer. They may take their first

steps, but don't expect this to happen by age one on the dot. As healthcare professionals, we don't get too concerned about walking by the age of one.
- Fine motor skills: Your baby has a refined pincer grasp by now and might even attempt to construct a little tower of two blocks.
- Language: Most babies start to use pointing as part of their non-verbal communication, and they may start to use one or two specific words, in addition to 'Mama' and 'Dada'. For example, their version of a sibling's or pet's name. Or if they use a soother, they may have a word for it like 'dodo'. They have probably learned how to wave 'bye-bye'.
- Social: Your baby's problem-solving skills are increasing as well. They will take the lid off a container to remove objects that they know are inside.

And so, your baby is one! Moving around, pointing at things, using some words … it's hard to believe how much they have grown and developed in 12 months.

SLEEP

By six months, your baby will need 10 to 14 hours of sleep over a 24-hour period and most of that sleep will be at nighttime. Your baby will have at least one, but usually two, naps: one in the morning and one in the afternoon. Naps may last 30 minutes to 2 hours.

Some babies may sleep through the night by six months, but many will not. A bit like developmental milestones, it can be hard not to compare your baby's sleep to that of your friends' and relatives' babies. Just remember that every baby is unique and just because your baby's sleep may be developing at a different rate does not mean there is anything wrong with your baby's sleep pattern.

Big changes are going on in your baby's brain between 6 and 12 months. They are developing their circadian rhythm, meaning their brain now knows the difference between night and day. They are more alert during daylight and sleepier at night.

Your baby's brain is now developed enough to allow them to sleep for consolidated periods of time – up to eight hours. However, your baby may continue to wake during the night. There are lots of possible reasons for this:

- Hunger: Some babies still need a feed at night, especially under nine months. Growth spurts can temporarily increase hunger too.
- Teething: Teething discomfort can peak around this age, often causing unsettled nights. You might notice flushed cheeks, extra drooling, or chewing.
- Separation anxiety: From around eight months, babies begin to understand that you can be away from them – and they don't like it. This can cause frequent waking, especially if they fell asleep with you nearby.
- Sleep associations: If your baby is used to being rocked, fed, or cuddled to sleep, they may struggle to get back to sleep on their own when they stir during the night.
- Developmental leaps: Major milestones, such as crawling, pulling up, or babbling, can disrupt sleep. Babies often 'practise' these new skills in their cot! It is really cute, but it can cause quite a bit of disruption in a home!
- Illness or discomfort: Colds, ear infections, or even a mild change in routine can interrupt sleep. If your baby is waking unusually often or seems unwell, check with your GP or public-health nurse.

Moving room

Now that your baby is getting older, you might be thinking about moving them into a room of their own. I had a hard time with this on my first baby. First, I couldn't bring myself to do it until she was about nine months old, then she just would not settle in her own room. Looking back, there are some things I would have done differently. For example, by waiting until she was nine months old, I hit the exact time she was starting to feel separation anxiety. So, it wasn't a great experience for any of us, unfortunately. Here are some tips I used the second time around!

- Choose the right time: Consider making the move when your baby is able to sleep for longer stretches at night. Avoid making the transition during times of upheaval, such as teething, illness, or holidays – or when they start to show signs of separation anxiety!
- Start with naps: Begin by letting your baby nap in their cot in the new room during the day. This helps them get used to the new environment while it's still light and less intimidating.
- Make the room comfortable: Ensure the room is a safe, cosy space. Use blackout blinds, keep the temperature comfortable (about 16–20°C is ideal), and maintain a calm atmosphere.
- Stick to your routine: A consistent bedtime routine, such as a bath, story, and cuddle, offers security and signals it's time for sleep, regardless of where they are.
- Use a monitor, and don't hover: A reliable baby monitor can offer reassurance without you needing to be in the room. Remember that it's okay to give your baby a moment to resettle themselves before going in.

You may decide you don't want to move your baby out of the room just yet, and that is fine too. All families are different; all babies are different. As long as you and your baby are getting enough sleep and feeling rested, do what works for you.

SKIN

By six months, you have probably settled into a skincare routine with your baby. However, eczema can still develop, as can nappy rash. See Chapter 4 (pages 88–90) for tips on how to manage these common skin conditions.

ILLNESSES AND ACCIDENTS

Illnesses

Between 6 and 12 months, your baby will start to interact with more people and possibly enter a crèche, daycare or childminding environment, thereby coming into contact with more non-family members – and that means more germs!

The illnesses babies of this age encounter are the same as those described in Chapter 4 (pages 95–103). Most of the illnesses will be viral, but some will be bacterial. Refer to pages 96 and 102 for the red flags of illnesses in babies.

Accidents

Your baby is also increasingly mobile, which raises the possibility of accidents. Even with the most thorough babyproofing in the world, accidents can still happen. And now that your baby is eating and also experimenting with putting non-food objects in their mouth, choking is a possibility.

Babyproofing

Here are some tips on babyproofing your home:

- Never leave your baby unattended on raised surfaces, such as changing tables, sofas, or beds, even for a few seconds.

- Use changing tables with safety straps and keep one hand on your baby at all times.
- Install safety gates at the top and bottom of stairs. Choose ones that screw into the wall for better security.
- Keep floors clear of clutter, especially small objects or slippery rugs that can trip an adult carrying a baby.
- Anchor heavy furniture, such as bookcases and TVs, to the wall to prevent them tipping over if your baby uses them to pull themselves up.
- Avoid placing baby bouncers, car seats, or rockers on raised surfaces – they can tip or slide off.
- Use window locks or restrictors. Both upstairs and downstairs windows should be baby-safe.
- Choose high chairs and baby seats with a five-point harness and always buckle your baby in securely.
- Avoid baby walkers as they increase the risk of falls down stairs and tip-overs, and they are of no benefit to a baby's walking skills.

Building confidence: take a first-aid course

One of the most empowering things a parent can do is attend a baby-specific first-aid class. Courses are widely available in both Ireland and the UK through trusted organisations, such as the British Red Cross, St John Ambulance, and the Irish Red Cross. Many offer in-person and online options, and some are even free of charge.

It is worth attending a baby first-aid course to equip yourself with the skills to deal with your newly mobile baby, but some of the basics are covered in the rest of this chapter.

Choking first aid

Choking occurs when something blocks your baby's airway, making it difficult or impossible for them to breathe. This can happen very quickly and may be silent, so it's essential to know what to look out for.

Warning signs your baby may be choking:

- struggling to cough or breathe
- no sound or very weak sounds when crying
- red or blue colouring in the face
- look of panic or distress
- flared nostrils or bulging eyes
- limp or unresponsive.

If your baby is coughing forcefully, allow them to try to clear the obstruction on their own. Do not place your fingers in your baby's mouth if they are coughing – you might cause them to inhale the object further.

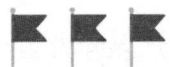

If your baby is silent, cannot cry, or begins to change colour, this is an emergency and immediate action is required.

WHAT TO DO IF YOUR BABY IS CHOKING

Call for help immediately if possible.

If there are other people in the house, yell for help at the top of your voice. If you are alone with your baby, start first aid (see steps on the next page and more detail on pages 311–315), but if the initial five back blows and five chest thrusts have not worked, call 999/112 and place your phone on speaker.

If you are alone and have no phone, consider running outside with baby, continuing first aid and yelling for help. I know this sounds dramatic but, in a situation like this, you will need help.

120 | SHOULD I BE WORRIED?

If you suspect your baby is choking and they cannot breathe or make any noise, immediately follow the first-aid steps listed below for a baby under age one.

Step 1: Check their mouth

- You should only remove the object with your fingers if you can clearly see it at the front of the mouth. Do not attempt to blindly sweep their mouth with your finger, as this can push the object deeper.

Step 2: Give five back blows

- Lay your baby face down along your forearm, supporting their head and jaw.
- Position their body so it is angled down towards the floor.
- Use the heel of your hand to give five sharp, firm back blows between the shoulder blades.

Step 3: Give five chest thrusts

- Turn your baby face up, resting them on your thigh or forearm.
- Place two fingers just below the nipple line, in the centre of the chest.
- Push inwards and upwards firmly but gently five times.
- Continue alternating five back blows and five chest thrusts until the object is expelled or help arrives.

If you have not already called the emergency services and your baby becomes unresponsive at any point, call 999/112 immediately and begin CPR (see CPR guidelines on pages 315–316).

Preventing choking: foods to avoid in the first year

Babies under one year are still learning to chew and swallow, and their airways are especially small. It's important to avoid giving them foods that are round, hard, sticky, or difficult to chew.

Avoid the following foods:

- whole grapes or cherry tomatoes (cut into quarters if given)
- raw, hard vegetables (e.g. carrots – always steam until soft)
- whole nuts and popcorn
- large chunks of meat or cheese (serve finely shredded or chopped)
- sausages or hot dogs (slice into thin strips lengthwise)
- marshmallows and chewy sweets
- thick dollops of peanut butter (spread thinly or mix into food)
- hard-boiled sweets or chewing gum.

Also, ensure your baby is seated upright and supervised during every meal or snack. Avoid letting them eat while lying back or crawling.

Hidden hazards: non-food choking risks in the home

It's not just food that poses a choking risk; babies love to put things in their mouths to explore, and many everyday household items can be dangerous.

A good rule of thumb is, if it fits through a toilet-roll tube, it's a choking hazard. Common non-food choking hazards are:

- button batteries (especially dangerous if swallowed)
- coins
- small toy parts, LEGO pieces, and board-game tokens
- beads, buttons, and jewellery

- pen caps
- deflated balloons or burst balloon pieces
- screws or plastic fittings from furniture
- pet food (dry kibble is especially risky).

Make a habit of getting down on the floor at baby level to scan for small items, especially after guests have visited or older siblings have been playing.

What about anti-choking devices?

In recent years, anti-choking suction devices have become more widely marketed, including for use with babies and children. These devices aim to dislodge objects by creating suction over the mouth and nose.

But are they safe for babies? The short answer: use with caution, and only as a last resort.

Irish and UK first-aid guidance does not currently recommend these devices as part of standard baby first aid, and research on them is limited. As of 2025, peer-reviewed, independent studies on the effectiveness and safety of these devices in infants are sparse. Most available evidence comes from case reports submitted by the manufacturers.

Some manufacturers claim their device can be used on babies over 10 kilograms (22 pounds), which does not include all infants under one year of age. There are also potential risks in using these devices:

- Improper use could cause injury to delicate baby tissues, especially in smaller infants.
- Delays in starting back blows and chest thrusts while using the device could worsen outcomes.
- Devices may not create effective suction on a baby's small, soft facial features.

Bottom line: if you choose to have an anti-choking device at home, treat it as a backup, not a replacement for knowing basic baby first aid.

> **WHEN IT COMES TO CHOKING, IN SUMMARY:**
> - Supervise your baby during meals and play.
> - Avoid or modify high-risk foods.
> - Learn the signs of choking and how to respond.
> - Consider a baby first-aid course for extra confidence and peace of mind.
> - Use anti-choking devices only if trained and only after first aid has failed.

First aid for falls

No matter how vigilant a parent may be, accidents can still happen, especially during the first year of life when babies are learning to roll, sit, and crawl. Falls are among the most common cause of injury in babies under one, and knowing how to respond can make all the difference.

What is a dangerous height?

Generally, a fall from a height greater than your baby's own height (around 2 feet or 60 centimetres) can be considered potentially dangerous. Falls from furniture, such as beds, sofas, changing tables, or down stairs carry a higher risk of injury, especially if the baby lands on a hard surface, such as tiled or wood flooring.

Particularly concerning are falls from:

- a height greater than 1 metre (e.g. off a kitchen counter or from a parent's arms)
- a baby carrier or car seat dropped from standing height
- staircases (especially tumbling down several steps).

Common injuries from falls

The most frequent injuries from falls include:

- minor bumps and bruises
- lumps on the head (also called 'goose eggs'), usually due to swelling under the scalp
- cuts or abrasions
- fractures, especially of the arm or collarbone
- mild concussions.

Less commonly, more serious injuries can occur, such as:

- skull fractures
- internal bleeding (e.g. within the brain)
- spinal injuries.

How you respond depends on how the baby is behaving after the fall and what kind of injury you suspect. Here's a guide to knowing what to do and when.

Call your GP (or out-of-hours GP) if:

- your baby has a bump on their head but is alert, feeding well, and acting normally
- there's mild bruising or a small cut that doesn't need stitches
- you're unsure whether the baby needs to be seen, but there are no obvious signs of serious injury.

Your GP can assess whether your baby needs to be seen in person or monitored at home.

Take your baby to the emergency department if they have any of these symptoms:

- they fall from a height greater than 1 metre
- they lose consciousness, even briefly
- they vomit more than once after the fall
- they are unusually drowsy or hard to wake
- they seem confused or dazed
- they have a seizure or convulsion
- there is any blood or clear fluid coming from their nose or ears
- they are not using one arm or leg, or seem to be in significant pain
- you notice swelling, deformity, or bruising that suggests a broken bone
- they fall down the stairs.

Always trust your instincts. If something feels off, it's worth getting checked.

Call 999/112 for an ambulance if:

- your baby is unconscious or unresponsive
- they are having a seizure
- they are not breathing properly or you're struggling to assess their breathing
- there is a suspected serious head, neck, or spinal injury (e.g. after a high fall)
- the baby is floppy, very pale, or hard to wake.

Even if your baby seems fine initially, keep a close eye on them for the next 24–48 hours.

Key things to monitor closely after a fall include:

- unusual sleepiness (beyond normal napping)
- changes in feeding patterns
- excessive crying or irritability
- balance or co-ordination issues (age-appropriate)
- persistent vomiting
- an enlarging or soft swelling on the scalp.

If any of these signs develop, seek medical advice promptly.

Most baby falls, though frightening, result in minor injuries. Even the most careful parents experience accidents. If your baby falls, try not to panic or blame yourself; instead, focus on your baby's behaviour and follow the advice on the previous pages. Seeking help quickly when needed is the best thing you can do.

FIRST AID FOR BURNS AND SCALDS IN INFANTS

In babies under 12 months, even a small burn or scald can have serious consequences. Their skin is thinner and more delicate than an adult's, meaning hot liquids or surfaces can cause deeper injuries in just a second.

If your baby is burned or scalded, follow these steps:

Step 1: Remove the heat source

- Gently take your baby away from the hot object or liquid. If clothing is wet with a hot liquid, remove it unless it's stuck to the skin. Remember to remove the nappy as it may have absorbed hot liquid.

Step 2: Cool the area immediately

- Hold the affected area under cool (not cold) running water for 20 minutes. If that's difficult – for example, if the burn or scald is on the face – use a clean cloth soaked in cool water and refresh it regularly.

Step 3: Do not use creams or ointments

- Avoid creams and ointments, as well as butter, ice, toothpaste, or other home remedies as they can worsen the damage.

Step 4: Cover the burn

- Use cling film – or, if you don't have any, a clean plastic nappy bag – to loosely cover the area. This helps reduce pain and prevent infection.

Step 5: Keep your baby warm and calm

- After running cool water over the burn for 20 minutes, wrap your baby in a blanket (avoiding the burn area), hold them close, and speak soothingly. Babies pick up on your anxiety, and your calm reassurance goes a long way.

Step 6: Seek medical attention straightaway

- Always get medical help for a baby under one with a burn or scald, no matter how small it looks. Contact your GP or out-of-hours service. Dial 999/112 if the face, hands, feet, genitals, or joints are involved.

Common causes of burns and scalds

At this age, babies don't understand danger, but they're often wriggly, curious, and love to reach and grab. Many burns in this age group happen in seconds, usually when parents are distracted just briefly.

Here are key hazards to be aware of:

- hot drinks on low tables or held while a caregiver is having a cuppa – even tea or coffee left to cool for 10–15 minutes can still cause serious scalds
- kettle cords dangling from the counter
- bath water that's too hot or running water left unattended
- radiators and heaters that babies can crawl or roll into
- hair straighteners, curling tongs, or irons left within reach
- microwaved baby food or milk – uneven heating can cause hotspots that burn your baby's mouth.

Key babyproofing tips to prevent burns and scalds

In the kitchen
- Use the back rings on the hob and turn pan handles towards the wall.
- Keep hot drinks away from edges, and never drink one while holding your baby.
- Fit oven-door locks and stove-knob covers if needed.
- Use a cord shortener for kettles and other countertop appliances.
- Feed warm drinks and food to baby with caution, ensuring they are not too hot.
- Don't microwave baby food or milk to heat it up.

In the bathroom
- Check the bath-water temperature every time before putting your baby in the water – it should ideally be around 37°C. Use a bath thermometer or your elbow as a guide. It should feel the same temperature as your elbow (this is very approximate!).
- Turn on the cold water first and off last when filling the bath.
- Keep your baby within arm's reach at all times; even a few seconds away can be enough time for an accident to happen.

Around the house
- Fit fireguards around open fires and radiators.
- Keep heated hair tools well out of reach and store them immediately after use.
- Avoid using tablecloths or runners where your baby might pull them down.

CONGRATULATIONS!

Now that your baby is one, you can look back with pride at the amazing job you have done so far. Can you believe that this little person has been in your life for 12 whole months?

In some ways, it may feel like your life has changed in an instant but, in others, you probably can't even remember or imagine life without this wonderful baby of yours. And now they are about to become a toddler.

Let the adventures begin!

CHAPTER 6
1 to 2 Years

At some point in the next six months, your baby is probably going to take their first steps (if they haven't already) and transform from a baby into a toddler. Are you ready? This is going to be fun – chaos, but fun!

FEEDING

By the age of one, your baby will be getting most of their nutrition from solid food, and, when they turn one, they can switch from formula to cow's milk (as long as they don't have a cow's-milk allergy or intolerance). If breastfeeding, you may also choose to wean them from breast to cow's milk. As your baby grows into toddlerhood, they might become opinionated about lots of things, and that includes food! This is a common age for 'picky' or 'fussy' eating to emerge.

Switching from formula to cow's milk

Guidelines recommend introducing full-fat cow's milk as a main drink from 12 months of age. Before this age, babies' kidneys aren't mature enough to process cow's milk efficiently, and it doesn't provide the right balance of nutrients, particularly iron, for infants under one.

After 12 months, you can begin offering cow's milk as a drink, while continuing to provide a varied diet that includes iron-rich foods, such as meat, lentils, green leafy vegetables, and fortified cereals.

How quickly can we make the switch?

You can make a direct switch to cow's milk at 12 months if your child is healthy and eating a good range of solid foods. There's no strict need to gradually wean off formula if your baby tolerates cow's milk well.

However, some parents choose to transition more slowly to help their child adjust to the new taste and consistency. A gradual switch might include:

- replacing one bottle of formula a day with cow's milk
- mixing cow's milk and formula together in increasing ratios.

Some tips for a smooth transition to cow's milk include:

- Use full-fat milk (whole milk) until at least age two, unless advised otherwise by your GP.
- Offer cow's milk in a cup, not a bottle, to encourage healthy oral habits.
- Limit cow's milk to around 350–400 millilitres per day. Too much can reduce iron absorption and appetite for solid foods.

Continue offering iron-rich meals to prevent iron deficiency, which is a common concern during the toddler years.

When to seek advice

If your child has a history of cow's-milk-protein allergy or intolerance, or if you have concerns about their nutrition, it's best to speak with a GP or public-health nurse before making any changes.

Switching from formula to cow's milk is a straightforward step for most families. While follow-on formula might seem like a helpful bridge, it's not needed if your child eats well.

When to get rid of the bottle

Hands up! Both of my children had a bedtime bottle until they were around two years old. That does not make me a 'bad' mum, and, if your little one gets comfort from a bottle, you should do what works best for you and your family. However, there are some advantages to dropping the bottle after the age of one.

It benefits your toddler's teeth if you drop the bottle early. Prolonged bottle use, especially when filled with milk or juice, can lead to tooth decay. This condition, often referred to as 'bottle mouth' or 'early-childhood caries', occurs when sugars from the liquid cling to the teeth for extended periods, particularly during naps and bedtime. Switching to a cup reduces this risk and encourages proper oral hygiene from an early age. Unfortunately, my tardiness in getting rid of the bottle for both of my kids probably did contribute to some dental decay and, if I had my time back again, I would have binned the bottles much earlier!

Toddlers who drink too much milk from a bottle often feel too full to eat solid foods. This can lead to nutritional imbalances, such as iron deficiency, because milk lacks key nutrients that are found in a varied diet. Transitioning from a bottle to a cup helps children to eat a range of healthy foods.

Continuing with bottles for prolonged periods can also affect speech development. Sucking on a bottle requires different muscle movements than drinking from a cup. When toddlers continue to use bottles, they may miss out on developing the oral motor skills necessary for proper speech and eating. Cups, especially those with straws or open tops, encourage stronger tongue, lip, and jaw co-ordination.

Ear infections are an unexpected side-effect of prolonged

bottle use. Bottle feeding while lying down can cause milk to flow into the Eustachian tubes, which increases the risk of ear infections. Cup drinking, particularly while seated upright, minimises this issue and supports overall ear health.

Letting go of the bottle is a positive step towards toddlerhood. While some resistance is normal, most children adjust within a few weeks with gentle consistency and encouragement.

Picky eating

The 'picky eating' phase can be stressful to navigate and I went through it with one of my children but not the other, which goes to show that all children are unique. Calling it 'picky eating' might seem to trivialise it, especially when you are in the throes of it, because as parents and caregivers we feel it is our job to feed and nourish our kids, and it can be really tough when our best efforts are rejected by them.

So, why do some toddlers become 'picky' eaters?

- Developmental stage: At around one to three years old, toddlers begin asserting their independence. Saying 'no' is a powerful tool for exerting control, and food is an easy area to do just that. A toddler's appetite also naturally decreases after their first year of rapid growth, which can make them more selective.
- Sensory issues: Young children are often more sensitive to textures, smells, and flavours. A mushy banana, a strong-smelling cheese, or a new texture in their mouth can be overwhelming. Some toddlers are more prone to sensory aversions than others.
- Fear of new foods (neophobia): It's common for toddlers to show fear or suspicion of unfamiliar foods. This tendency is actually thought to have an evolutionary purpose – it protects us from eating potentially harmful substances.
- Parental pressure: It's natural to worry if your child is eating

'enough', but pressuring or bribing toddlers to eat can backfire. Children may become even more resistant when they feel coerced.

Strategies for managing picky eating

The key to managing picky eating in toddlers is to maintain a calm, consistent approach while creating a positive food environment. Establishing a regular routine is helpful. Aim to serve three balanced meals and two healthy snacks at roughly the same times each day. Avoid letting your toddler graze between meals, as this can dull their appetite and reduce their interest in trying new foods.

It's also a good idea to prepare just one meal for the whole family, rather than offering alternatives to suit your toddler's preferences. This not only eases the pressure on you, but also reinforces the idea that mealtimes are shared and not subject to negotiation. When you serve food, include at least one familiar item you know your child usually eats, alongside any new or less preferred foods. Encourage your toddler to explore what's on offer, but don't force them to eat. Repeated gentle exposure without pressure is often what eventually leads to acceptance.

Your own eating habits can have a big impact too. Toddlers are keen observers, and they learn by watching you. Sitting down to eat the same food with enthusiasm can model positive behaviour and make new foods seem more approachable. Try to keep mealtimes relaxed and free from conflict. If your child refuses to eat, resist the urge to bribe or negotiate; simply remove the plate after a reasonable time and carry on with your routine.

Involving your toddler in preparing food can also boost their interest. Even simple tasks like stirring ingredients, washing vegetables, or helping to set the table give them a sense of ownership and curiosity about the meal. This can reduce anxiety and make them more open to trying the food they've helped create.

One widely recommended approach is the 'division of responsibility' in feeding. This means that as the parent, you decide what food is offered, when it is offered, and where it is served. Your child, in turn, gets to decide whether to eat it and how much they eat. This shared responsibility helps avoid power struggles and enables your toddler to listen to their own hunger and fullness cues.

When to seek help

Picky eating is usually a normal phase. However, speak to your GP or public-health nurse if:

- your child is losing weight or dropping centiles on their growth chart
- they consistently refuse entire food groups
- you suspect sensory-processing issues or chewing difficulties
- mealtimes are a constant source of anxiety or distress.

GROWTH

Remember the old days when your baby doubled their weight between birth and six months? Well, those days are no more! Your toddler will gain about 2–3 kilograms over the next 12 months, at a rate of 50–100 grams per week. Their height will increase by 10–12 centimetres.

At 18-months, the average boy weighs 10.9 kilograms and measures 82.5 centimetres, and the average girl weighs 10.6 kilograms and measures 81 centimetres. The average calorie requirement for 12-to-24-month-olds is 1,000–1,400 calories per day, usually taken as three main meals and two to three snacks.

Faltering growth

If you notice that your toddler is not gaining weight or is losing weight, you should get them reviewed by your GP. There are lots of possible reasons for faltering growth in this age group. If they are going through a phase of picky eating, they may not be consuming enough calories to support growth. If they are eating well but not growing, their ability to absorb food may be impaired.

Coeliac disease, which is a reaction to gluten, can present in this age group. The gut becomes inflamed and damaged as a result of the reaction to gluten and nutrients from food that are not properly absorbed. Signs of coeliac disease include poor weight gain, weight loss, tummy bloating, constipation or diarrhoea, and irritability. Your doctor can request a blood test that screens for coeliac disease and may refer your toddler to a paediatrician for further tests and treatment.

DEVELOPMENTAL MILESTONES

Toddlerhood is a time of big developmental leaps, but not all toddlers develop at the same rate and many develop certain skills at faster rates than others. For example, you may have a 17-month-old who is not walking independently but who is talking in short sentences, or a 15-month-old who has been walking since the age of 10 months but has very few words. Remember, milestones are just a tool to help healthcare professionals identify signs of developmental delay at an early stage and facilitate early intervention. If you have competitive parents in your vicinity, tune them out. Focus on your own unique and fabulous toddler.

Here are some milestones we look out for between the ages of 13 and 24 months.

Gross motor skills

Most toddlers are learning to walk during this time and many will be moving confidently by 15 months. At first, walking may be wobbly with frequent tumbles, but you'll notice them getting stronger and steadier week by week. As they grow in confidence, they'll start climbing onto furniture, crawling up stairs (with supervision), and pulling toys behind them as they walk.

By around 18 months, some toddlers will try to run, walk backwards, or even kick a ball, although co-ordination is still a work in progress! By 24 months, many children are running more smoothly, climbing onto furniture without hesitation, and starting to jump with both feet off the ground. They're becoming stronger and more co-ordinated.

Fine motor skills

When it comes to hand skills and vision, your child will begin to use their fingers more precisely. By this age, toddlers can pick up small objects using a neat pincer grasp and will love putting things in and out of containers.

Many will enjoy turning pages in board books and may attempt to scribble with crayons. You may start to notice a preference for one hand or the other by 13–14 months, indicating whether your toddler might be right-handed or left-handed.

Around 16 to 18 months, toddlers often begin stacking blocks, pointing to pictures in books, and trying to use a spoon or drink from an open cup. As they approach their second birthday, their hands become more skilful. They might turn doorknobs, build taller block towers, and use a spoon or fork with more control, although spills are still common. You may also see them start to help with dressing by taking off hats, shoes, or socks, and showing interest in zips and buttons.

Language

Language development is also rapidly progressing. Even if your toddler isn't saying many words just yet, they're likely to understand far more than you think. By 13–15 months, many children will say a few simple words beyond 'Mama' or 'Dada' and begin to follow easy instructions like, 'Give me the ball.' They'll use gestures, such as pointing, waving, or shaking their head, and their babble may start to sound more like real conversation.

As your child approaches 18 months, their vocabulary often expands to include 10–20 words, and some toddlers may start putting two words together, such as 'more milk' or 'bye, Mama'. By 24 months, many toddlers will have 50 or more words and will start combining two or more words into short phrases, such as 'want juice' or 'Mama go work'. They also understand much more than they can say and will often follow two-step instructions, such as, 'Pick up your toy and put it in the box.'

Social and emotional

Socially and emotionally, toddlers are developing stronger bonds and preferences. You may notice they become clingier or more wary of strangers, which is a normal part of growing attachment. They might hand you a book to read or copy your everyday activities in their play. Although they're still mostly playing alongside rather than with other children (known as 'parallel play'), they're increasingly aware of others and show a growing desire to connect and communicate.

You'll also see more emotional reactions (joy, frustration, pride, and, sometimes, full-blown tantrums) as your child learns to navigate their feelings. Simple pretend play becomes more sophisticated too: your child might feed a doll, pretend to drive a car, or mimic your daily routines. By two years old, many children show signs of independence, such as wanting to feed themselves and help with simple tasks, or even insist on doing things 'all by myself'.

Cognitively, toddlers become like little scientists. They might experiment with cause and effect: dropping objects to see what happens or repeatedly opening and closing containers. You'll likely find them trying to open cupboards, stack toys, or imitate what they see you do. Their memory and understanding of routines strengthens, and they may even start to anticipate what comes next in familiar situations, like bath time or bedtime.

Whilst there is a wide range of what is 'typical' for developmental milestones in this age group, there are a few signs worth keeping an eye on. It is worth speaking to your GP or public-health nurse for advice if:

- your child is not walking by 18 months
- they do not respond to their name
- they are not using gestures like pointing or waving
- they have not started saying any words.

Early support is important to help your toddler reach their developmental milestones if they are showing delay in some areas.

SLEEP

As your toddler's brain develops, their sleep pattern changes. A 12-to-24-month-old needs 12–15 hours of sleep in 24 hours, broken into 10–12 hours of sleep at night and 2–3 hours of napping during the day. In this period, your toddler may transition from a morning and afternoon nap to a single afternoon nap.

Your toddler may still not be sleeping through the night. Although a 13-month-old toddler can physically sleep through without needing to wake for milk, this does not mean that they can manage a full 10–12 hours without waking.

Why are they still waking?

There are several reasons why your toddler might not be sleeping through the night, even if they once did.

- Separation anxiety: One of the most common reasons is separation anxiety, which often peaks between 12 and 18 months. Your child is beginning to understand that you exist even when you're not in the room, and that awareness can bring with it a fear of being apart, especially at night.
- Teething: The molars often start to come in during this stage and, for some children, that means sore gums and disrupted sleep.
- Developmental milestones: Toddlers are also busy reaching new developmental milestones, including learning to walk, talk, and assert their independence. All this brain and body development can cause nighttime restlessness.
- Sleep associations: These can play a role too. If your child falls asleep every night being rocked or fed, they may struggle to resettle without the same help when they wake in the night. These associations can become quite strong by this age, so breaking them takes patience and consistency.
- Change in routine: Any changes to their routine, such as illness, travel, or even starting crèche, can knock sleep off course. These disruptions are usually temporary, although they can feel never-ending when you're up at 3 am for the fourth night in a row.

How can you help?

Consistency is key. Establishing a simple, calming bedtime routine helps signal to your child that it's time to wind down. This might include a warm bath, a couple of quiet stories, and some relaxed time in their darkened room before sleep.

Try to put your toddler down when they're sleepy but still

awake. This gives them the chance to fall asleep on their own, which can make it easier for them to self-settle if they wake during the night.

If your child is waking due to teething or discomfort, speak to your GP about safe pain-relief options. A favourite teddy or blanket can also offer comfort and security during unsettled nights, especially if separation anxiety is in play.

When they do wake, keep interactions calm and brief. Offer reassurance, but try not to start the bedtime routine all over again. Some parents find a gentle approach, such as gradually reducing how much they soothe their child, works well, while others feel more comfortable staying nearby until their child nods off again. Trust your instincts and choose what feels right for your family.

When to ask for help

If sleep challenges are affecting your child's mood during the day or your own well-being is taking a hit, don't hesitate to ask for help. Your GP can rule out any medical causes and your public-health nurse can advise you on sleep support if needed.

VACCINES

Let's talk about the vaccination schedule for toddlers aged 12–18 months and the diseases these vaccines prevent. Remember that, if at any stage you have questions about the vaccines that are offered, you can speak to your GP or public-health nurse, who will be able to give you helpful and factual information.

Vaccines administered at 12 months

- MMR: Protects against measles, mumps and rubella. Measles can cause pneumonia, brain inflammation, and death. It is highly contagious. On average, one in four

children who get measles will need to be hospitalised. Mumps can lead to meningitis, deafness, and, in rare cases, infertility. Rubella is usually mild but it is dangerous during pregnancy, where it can cause serious problems for the foetus, such as congenital rubella syndrome, which is associated with deafness, blindness, and cardiac complications.
- MenB: Protects against Meningococcal B, which is a major cause of bacterial meningitis in children. The disease can progress rapidly and is often fatal or severely disabling.
- Chickenpox: As of autumn 2025, the varicella vaccine has been added to to the national childhood immunisation schedule in Ireland. It has been part of the vaccination schedule in the USA since 1995, and is now part of the schedule in Canada, Australia, and New Zealand.

Vaccines administered at 13 months

- Hib/MenC: Protects against Hib (Haemophilus influenzae type b), which can cause meningitis, pneumonia, and epiglottitis (severe swelling and obstruction of the airway), and MenC (Meningococcal C), which can cause meningitis and septicaemia, with a risk of death or long-term complications.
- Pneumococcal (PCV): Protects against Streptococcus pneumoniae, which causes pneumonia, meningitis, and blood infections.

Side-effects and how to help your child

While vaccines are safe and closely monitored, mild side-effects can occur. These usually appear within 24–48 hours.
Common reactions include:

- mild fever
- soreness or swelling at the injection site

- irritability or sleepiness
- loss of appetite.

With the MenB vaccine, fever is more common. Paracetamol (appropriate for your child's age and weight) is often recommended just prior to getting the vaccine to reduce discomfort and fever. Check with your GP if they are happy for you to go ahead and do this.

If your child does have a reaction to a vaccine, you can help by:

- offering cuddles and reassurance
- keeping them cool and hydrated
- giving them paracetamol or ibuprofen as advised
- letting them rest and take it easy for the day.

If a high fever lasts more than 48 hours or you are concerned about your child's reaction, contact your GP.

Vaccine hesitancy

I have already spoken about vaccine hesitancy and its history on page 74, but it is worth reiterating here that scientific research consistently shows that vaccines are safe and effective. They are rigorously tested before approval and continuously monitored for safety. Vaccines play a vital role in protecting your baby from illnesses that can have severe or life-threatening consequences.

Reactions to vaccines are generally mild and temporary, whereas the diseases they prevent are often severe and, in some cases, deadly. Choosing to vaccinate is a step towards protecting your child during their early years.

If you have concerns, speaking to your GP or public-health nurse can provide reassurance and clear information.

The difference between misinformation (false but shared in

error) and disinformation (deliberately misleading) is important. Seek trusted sources like:

- In Ireland, HSE (hse.ie)
- In the UK, NHS (nhs.uk)
- World Health Organization (who.int)
- GP or public-health nurse.

ACCIDENTS AND ILLNESSES

I mentioned the possibility of your child getting a 'goose egg' bump in Chapter 5, and if you are not familiar with them by now, it is highly likely that your toddler will acquire one in the next 12 months or so. Tumbles, bumps, and bruises are part and parcel of life now that your toddler is toddling, climbing, maybe trying to run, and still developing a sense of what is safe and what is not.

By now, no doubt, your house will be toddler-proofed, but you won't always be in your house and accidents will happen despite your best efforts to prevent them. If you haven't taken a baby and toddler first-aid course, now might be the time to look into one.

Falls

Having worked in hospitals around Ireland, and indeed around the world, I have seen the most incredible, unanticipated accidents befall toddlers. But the most common reason toddlers end up in the emergency department with an injury is falls.

Most often, these falls result in nothing more than bruises or the occasional bump (those famous goose eggs!) to the forehead. Parents understandably worry about head injuries, but the good news is that most minor head bumps in toddlers don't lead to serious problems. If your child cries immediately, is consolable, and returns to their normal behaviour within a short time, there's usually little to worry about. But if you are in any doubt, get your toddler checked out.

The following are some red flags for head injury. You should attend the emergency department for a head injury if:

- the fall was from more than 3 feet/1 metre or greater than your toddler's height
- there is a loss of consciousness, even briefly
- your child vomits more than once after the injury
- they have a seizure or convulsion
- they are unusually drowsy or you have difficulty waking them
- there is a weakness in or they have difficulty moving their arms or legs
- they have unequal pupil size or abnormal eye movements
- there is clear fluid or blood coming from the nose or ears
- they have slurred speech or confusion
- there is persistent crying or extreme irritability
- there is a soft, boggy swelling on the head.

Is it broken?

In this age group, bone fractures (or breaks) are not common, but they do happen, even after seemingly minor falls. The good news is that young children's bones tend to heal quickly. The important thing is knowing what to look out for, what to do when it happens, and when to seek help.

Sprains, strains and bruises can be managed at home with rest and pain relief. Fractures need to be managed in a hospital. This table will help you differentiate between a bump and a break but, if in doubt, get your toddler checked out!

SYMPTOM	FRACTURE	SPRAIN/STRAIN	BRUISE
Pain	Immediate, intense, persistent	Mild to moderate	May cry at first but settles
Swelling	Common, especially around joints	Common	Localised swelling is possible
Bruising	May develop after a few hours	Likely	Immediate or next day
Movement	Will refuse to use the limb or walk	May use the limb with discomfort	Uses limb normally after short rest
Touch	Cries or pulls away when area is touched	Mild discomfort	Tolerates touch
Deformity	May appear crooked or shorter	None	None

Listed here are the fractures we see most frequently in toddlers learning to walk, climb and run:

- Toddler's fracture (spiral fracture of the tibia): This often occurs without a dramatic-looking mechanism of injury. For example, a child might slip while running or twist a leg awkwardly while coming down a step. It's a tiny, hairline crack in the shinbone that doesn't always show up on X-rays straightaway. Often, the first clue is that they suddenly won't walk or they limp without an obvious bruise or swelling.
- Collarbone fracture (clavicle): This happens when a toddler falls directly onto their shoulder from a low chair, changing

table, or, sometimes, even from standing height. Your child may cry when picked up under the arms and avoid using one arm.
- Forearm fracture (radius/ulna): This usually occurs when a toddler has fallen onto their outstretched hand. Toddlers instinctively throw their hands forwards to break a fall. If they cry when you try to hold their hand or won't use the arm, this might be the cause.
- Supracondylar fracture (just above the elbow): This is a less common fracture but a more serious one. It happens due to a fall directly on the elbow or an outstretched arm, and it can affect circulation or nerves in the arm. This kind of fracture needs urgent attention.

Thankfully, most toddler fractures are simple and heal quickly. A soft cast or splint may be used for three to six weeks, and no surgery is needed in most cases. Bone remodelling in toddlers is excellent. Even slightly bent or misaligned bones often straighten themselves as the child grows.

If you suspect your toddler has a fracture, do the following:

- Reassure: Pick them up gently and try to calm them. Reassure them, and don't try to 'test' the limb too much.
- Immobilise: If it's an arm, you can create a makeshift sling using a tea towel or scarf. If it's a leg, try to limit movement and carry them.
- Apply ice: Wrap ice in a cloth and place it on the affected area for 10–15 minutes to reduce swelling.
- Pain relief: Paracetamol or ibuprofen is safe for toddlers, and it is okay to administer pain relief before leaving home if you are seeking medical attention.
- Seek medical advice: If they refuse to bear weight, won't move the limb, or you suspect a break, head to your nearest minor injuries unit or emergency department. X-rays may be needed and prompt care is important.

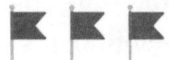

Below are some red flags for breaks and fractures. Call an ambulance if:

- the limb looks severely deformed or is pointing the wrong way
- your child is in extreme pain and cannot be moved safely
- the bone has broken through the skin
- there's numbness, pale or bluish skin, or no movement in the fingers or toes (this could signal circulation or nerve problems)
- your child has fallen from a significant height (more than their own height) and seems drowsy, confused, or very lethargic
- there are multiple injuries or you suspect a head injury, especially if there was loss of consciousness or vomiting.

PETER'S STORY

Peter was a typical 19-month-old boy: curious, energetic, and, in his parents' words, 'into everything'. When they heard a crash, they went running, only to find him at the bottom of the stairs. He had somehow opened the staircase and climbed the stairs, but lost his footing and tumbled all the way down. His mum checked to see if he was conscious and breathing. She could see his chest rising up and down, but he was unresponsive.

His dad called 999 and, when his call was answered, he was asked which service they wanted – fire, ambulance or coast guard. He requested 'ambulance' and was put through to the ambulance control centre. He explained what had happened and that Peter was unconscious. He was asked for their address and their Eircode. They were advised not to move Peter. They remained on the phone to the ambulance control centre until an advanced paramedic arrived at their house. Peter's dad shut the family dog safely into the living room and opened the front door.

Just as the paramedic arrived, Peter started to moan, but he did not open his eyes or seem aware of his parents. The paramedic set to work assessing Peter's condition and getting him ready for transfer to the ambulance, which arrived shortly afterwards. Peter's parents later recalled that the house seemed full of people, all gathered around their little boy.

Peter was blue-lighted to the nearest emergency department, with his mum in the ambulance with him and his dad driving behind. The paramedic had called ahead to the hospital and a full team were waiting in a room called the 'resus room' when Peter was brought into the emergency department. Tests, including X-rays and a CT scan of the brain, were done very quickly, and Peter's parents were told he had a brain bleed and needed urgent surgery. All they could do was wait.

I first met Peter two days later in the intensive-care unit. He looked so small in the bed, his head wrapped with a white bandage, bruising under both his eyes. But he was showing some promising signs of recovery. He was ready to start breathing by himself and, as the

> medications for sedation and pain relief were weaned, he started to open his eyes and recognise his parents.
>
> Peter's mum and dad were distraught. They blamed themselves for his accident. I assured them that they were not to blame and that accidents can happen in the blink of an eye, even when parents do everything 'right'.
>
> Peter made a full recovery and went home with his parents after about three weeks in hospital.
>
> Peter is, of course, a fictional amalgamation of the many toddlers I have met over the years with serious head injuries – and Peter had a happy ending.
>
> There are lots of reasons for toddlers to sustain a head injury, but the most common ones are falls, furniture tip-overs, and road-traffic collisions.

Common illnesses

In addition to being accident-prone during toddlerhood, you can also think of 12–24 months as the season of snot. Illness at this age can seem relentless, as your child meets countless new viruses that their immune system has to learn to deal with. I often meet parents who are exhausted, worried, and unsure whether their toddler's constant runny nose or cough is normal or something to worry about. So, here is a guide through the most common illnesses in this age group, and the warning signs that tell us a child might need more urgent medical help.

The common cold

You may feel like your toddler has a permanent cold, and, in many ways, they do! The average child under two can catch 8–12 viral infections a year. Runny noses, mild fevers, coughs, and clinginess are all normal. Most of the time, colds will pass with rest, hydration, and lots of cuddles. If they have a fever or sore throat, you can give paracetamol or ibuprofen. Over-the-counter cough medications and decongestants are not recommended for children under the age of six.

Ear infections

These can flare up quickly after a cold. You might notice your toddler tugging their ear, crying more at night, or having a fever. They often resolve on their own but, sometimes, antibiotics are needed, especially if symptoms persist beyond a couple of days or worsen. (See page 180 for more details on ear infections.) If your child has an ear infection, pain relief is very important, so give them regular paracetamol or ibuprofen.

Tummy upset

Gastroenteritis (vomiting and diarrhoea) is also very common, especially in crèche or nursery settings. The biggest risk isn't the bug itself, but dehydration. Offer fluids regularly, even in small sips, and make sure that your child is still peeing and not excessively sleepy or listless. Half-strength apple juice (half apple juice, half water) is a tasty option to help keep your little one hydrated. Oral rehydration solution (a special drink with electrolytes) can also be offered, but make sure you speak to your doctor or pharmacist to get advice before giving this. See page 337 for more detailed information on managing gastroenteritis.

Teething troubles

By this age, those molars may be starting to push through, often with more drama than the first teeth. Teething can make your toddler irritable, dribbly, and off their food. You might find that a dose of paracetamol or ibuprofen at nighttime helps with sleep. Offering cool foods at mealtimes can also be soothing. Your toddler's temperature might by slightly higher than normal, but shouldn't be more than 38°C. High fevers or prolonged diarrhoea are not caused by teething and should be investigated.

Croup, bronchiolitis, and chest infections

If your child has a barking cough (like a seal) or noisy breathing, it may be croup. This tends to sound worse at night and can be scary, but most cases are mild. Bronchiolitis can also cause coughing and wheezing, particularly in younger toddlers. You can read more about managing breathing problems in Chapter 15, from page 305. If your child is breathing very fast, using extra muscles to breathe, or not feeding, that's a red flag.

The following are some red flags to watch out for if your toddler is ill.

Fever red flags

- a temperature over 39°C in a child under two that doesn't respond to paracetamol or ibuprofen
- a fever lasting more than five days
- a fever with no obvious cause, especially if your child seems drowsy, hard to wake, or very irritable.

Breathing troubles

- breathing that is faster than usual, with chest sucking in or nostrils flaring
- a grunting sound when breathing out
- bluish lips or face
- a cough that causes your child to vomit, turn red, or struggle to catch their breath.

Dehydration signs

- fewer than three wet nappies in 24 hours
- a dry mouth, cracked lips, or no tears when crying
- unusual drowsiness or floppiness.

Rashes

- a non-blanching rash (one that doesn't fade when you press a glass against it) could be a sign of meningitis
- any rash accompanied by high fever, vomiting, or refusal to feed.

Neurological concerns

- seizures (especially ones lasting over five minutes or not linked to fever)
- new weakness in a limb, loss of balance, or your toddler refusing to walk when they previously could
- behaviour changes
- inconsolable crying where your toddler seems in pain and can't be soothed
- floppiness, listlessness, or extreme sleepiness.

If you have a concern about your toddler, even if they are not displaying any red flags, it is always best to speak to a healthcare professional or get them medically reviewed. Even the chattiest toddler will struggle to tell you exactly how they are feeling or where it hurts. It is better to get your child reviewed and to be told all is well than to be worrying at home that something is seriously wrong.

CONGRATULATIONS!

And now your toddler is two. In one year, they have transformed from a baby to a mobile, probably opinionated little character, who is starting to express their likes and dislikes. You will love them with all your heart, and they will love you right back!

CHAPTER 7
2 to 5 Years

Your little one is going to grow from being a toddler to a preschooler in these next three years. There are lots of thrills and spills ahead!

FEEDING

By now, your little one will probably be eating a wide range of foods. Phases of fussy or picky eating are also very normal in this age group. As your child tries more foods, there is also a small chance that they may have an allergic reaction. I describe allergies and anaphylaxis in detail on pages 85 and 297, but here's a recap of the signs of an allergic reaction:

Mild to moderate reactions:
- itchy mouth
- hives
- facial swelling
- tummy pain
- vomiting.

Severe reactions (anaphylaxis – call 999/112):
- difficulty breathing or noisy breathing
- sudden hoarse cry

- persistent cough
- pale or floppy
- swelling of tongue/throat
- collapse.

As your child grows, their nutritional requirements change. It doesn't seem that long ago when your little one got all the nutrition they needed from breast milk or infant formula. With increasing focus via social-media influencers on 'good' versus 'bad' foods for your child, and rising rates of children being overweight and obese, you might be feeling under pressure to get things 'right' with your toddler's or preschooler's nutrition.

I remember feeling this pressure intensely when my kids were aged three and five. I wanted to make sure they had the 'perfect' diet. They had other ideas! By that stage, they were spirited little humans with opinions and the ability to say 'no' to broccoli. In the end, I accepted that my kids' diet was something that would have to fall under the 'good enough' category as opposed to 'perfect' when it came to parenting. And guess what? As teenagers, broccoli is one of their absolute favourite foods. They say it reminds them of their childhood, which cracks me up!

When planning your little one's food for each day, you want to meet their basic requirements for calories, fats, proteins, carbohydrates (the macronutrients), fibre, and vitamins and minerals (the micronutrients).

That can seem like a big responsibility, but here is a breakdown of your child's nutritional needs:

- Protein: Supports growth, immune function, and muscle development.
- Carbohydrates: Provide essential energy.
- Fats: Crucial for brain development, vitamin absorption, and satiety (feeling full).

In general, your child's approximate calorie intake per day will be as follows:

Age	Calories†	Protein	Carbohydrates*	Total Fat	Fibre
2–3 years	1,000–1,400 kcal	13–20 g	At least 130 g	30–40% of kcal	15 g
4–5 years	1,200–1,600 kcal	14–22 g	At least 130 g	25–35% of kcal	15 g

† In relation to the figures in the table, note, however, that the calorie range varies with size and activity, so let your child's appetite guide you.
* Prioritise whole-grain breads, oats, potatoes with skin, and fruit and vegetables over sugary snacks.

Generally, your child will eat three meals over the course of a day, with two or three snacks. Typically, each meal will include a portion of each of the macronutrients (proteins, fats, carbohydrates) plus one or two portions of fruit and/or vegetables. But what is a 'portion' for a child? Thankfully, portions are pretty easy to measure – you can use your child's own hand as a guide, which grows with them, so you'll always get it right!

- Fruit/vegetables: child's cupped hand.
- Protein: child's palm.
- Carbohydrates: child's fist.
- Fats: thumb tip (about 5 millilitres).

Your child's three main meals will look something like this:

Macronutrient	Portions Per Meal	Example Portions
Protein	1 portion (occasionally 2 at dinner)	1 egg, child's palm of chicken/fish, 2 tablespoons lentils or beans, ½ matchbox tofu, 2 tablespoons hummus
Carbohydrates	1–2 portions	1 small slice wholemeal bread, ½–1 child's fist cooked rice/pasta/potato, 1 oatcake

Macronutrient	Portions Per Meal	Example Portions
Fats	1 portion (included or added)	1 teaspoon olive oil/butter, 1 teaspoon nut butter, 1 tablespoon grated cheese, ¼ avocado

And their snacks will look like this:

Macronutrient	Portions Per Snack	Example Portions
Protein or Fat	1 portion	Small cheese slice, yogurt (2–3 tablespoons), nut butter on toast, egg muffin
Carbohydrates	1 portion	Small banana, rice cake, oat biscuit, ½ slice toast, crackers

GROWTH

Between the ages of two and five, your toddler will gain approximately 6–7 kilograms in weight and grow about 20–25 centimetres.

Up until now, you will have been focused on making sure that your baby or young toddler has been getting enough food and been gaining enough weight. However, between the ages of two and five, parents sometimes become concerned that their child might be gaining *too much* weight. Conversations around being overweight and obesity are often emotionally charged because, as adults, discussions in this space can feel judgemental and stigmatising.

However, if you do have concerns about excessive weight gain in your child, they are important conversations to have with your GP or public-health nurse, because some simple measures can have beneficial effects on your child's current and future health.

Understanding being overweight

At this age, children grow in rapid, uneven spurts, so a round tummy or 'baby fat' is often normal. I used to joke that my kids always grew 'out' before they grew 'up'! To know whether any extra kilos are simply part of a growth phase or a genuine concern, you need objective growth data, not a visual guess.

A tall four-year-old will naturally weigh more than a shorter peer. Looking at weight-for-age alone might label the taller child 'overweight' when their weight is, in fact, appropriate for their height. Weight-for-height (BMI-for-age) corrects for this, giving a truer picture of proportional growth.

If you think your child is becoming overweight, book an appointment with your GP or raise your concern with the public-health nurse during your child's developmental checks. They will measure both height and weight, plot them on the centile charts, and explain where your child sits. If your child tracks above the 85th centile on weight-for-height and is not similarly high on height-for-age, that's the point to start gentle lifestyle changes.

Healthcare professionals look for trends over several months, so you may be asked to return in two to three months for repeat measurements before being advised on any further steps you may need to take to get your child's growth back on track.

Many parents feel guilty or blame themselves when they are told their child is overweight, but childhood weight gain is influenced by multiple factors: genetics, sleep, activity, food marketing, and more. You are not alone – and you are not a bad parent.

The key is to start early, be kind to yourself, and take a whole-family approach to healthy eating and activity. Remember, you are not putting your child on a 'diet' or trying to make them lose weight; the aim is to keep your child's weight steady while their height catches up. It is best to do this with input from your GP or public-health nurse, who may also advise review with a registered dietician.

Tips for food intake and activity levels

The following are the tips that you are likely to be given regarding your child's food and activity.

Avoid blame
It's important not to make your child feel like there is something wrong with their body. At this age, children are developing their self-image and food relationships.

Avoid focusing on weight
Instead of focusing on weight, frame changes as 'helping our family feel stronger and healthier'. Avoid terms like 'fat' or 'diet', and model healthy habits yourself. They are more likely to follow your lead than your words.

Reassess daily foods
You don't need to make drastic changes. Instead, focus on small, sustainable adjustments to your family's meals and snacks:

- Offer balanced meals: Half the plate for fruit and vegetables, a quarter for protein (lean meat, fish, eggs, beans), and a quarter for carbohydrates (rice, pasta, potatoes).
- Keep sugary foods occasional: Sweets, cakes, and crisps should be limited to special treats, not daily snacks.
- Watch portion sizes: Young children don't need adult-sized servings. Use child-sized plates and let them serve themselves when possible.
- Limit sugary drinks: Encourage your child to drink water and milk instead of juice or squash. Avoid fizzy drinks.

Encourage physical activity
Children aged two to five should be physically active for at least three hours a day, spread throughout the day. This doesn't have to be structured exercise. It can include:

- playing in the garden or park
- walking or scooting to crèche or preschool
- dancing to music at home
- climbing, jumping, or riding a trike.

Try to limit any screen time to no more than one hour a day, swapping some tablet or TV time for active play.

Work on their routine

Children thrive on routine: predictable mealtimes, consistent bedtimes, and regular snack schedules help regulate their appetite and energy. Avoid letting them graze all day, instead aim for three meals and two planned snacks.

You can also prioritise adequate sleep, as poor sleep is linked to increased weight gain. Toddlers need 11–14 hours of sleep per 24 hours; preschoolers need 10–13 hours.

Remember, you are not alone in this. There are high numbers of toddlers with weight issues around the world, and this is not an individual failing on the part of parents. There is help available to you and your child. Spotting excessive weight gain in your 2–5-year-old can feel worrying, but it's also a valuable opportunity. Early childhood is a period of rapid change, and small shifts taken now can lay the foundation for a lifetime of healthy habits.

What about supplements?

When you're the parent of a young child, it can feel like nutrition is a moving target. One week, your toddler adores spinach; the next, they eat only toast and yogurt. It's no wonder many parents consider vitamin supplements useful to fill in the nutritional gaps during those unpredictable phases.

Social media is full of cheerful influencers and promises that one chewable a day will solve every picky-eating worry. But do these supplements actually benefit young children? Could they cause harm?

In both Ireland and the UK, national health authorities make clear recommendations for this age group, based on common deficiencies, our climate, and the needs of growing bodies.

In the UK, children aged six months to five years are advised to take a daily supplement of vitamins A, C, and D, unless they are drinking more than 500 millilitres of infant formula a day (as this is already fortified). By the age of two, your toddler is unlikely to still be drinking infant formula.

In Ireland, the focus is on vitamin D. Children aged one to four are recommended to take 5 micrograms of vitamin D daily, especially between October and March when sunshine levels are low and natural synthesis is limited. These recommendations are based on the fact that many children in this age group do not get enough vitamin D through their food and sunlight, and that vitamins A and C may be lacking in fussy eaters.

What about multivitamins?

In general, healthy children who are eating a varied diet and taking the recommended vitamin D (or A/C/D) drops do not need an additional multivitamin. However, there are exceptions where a multivitamin may be useful:

- if your child has a highly restricted diet due to sensory issues, autism, or prolonged fussy eating
- if your child follows a vegan or medically restricted diet that excludes several food groups
- if your child is recovering from illness or surgery and their appetite is reduced.

In these situations, a multivitamin can provide short-term support. But it's important that any supplement you use matches the actual needs of your child and doesn't exceed safe limits for things such as vitamin A, iron, or zinc.

A chat with your GP, public-health nurse or pharmacist can help you choose the right product, if needed.

How about omega-3, probiotics, or other extras?

Some parents also ask about omega-3s, probiotics, or 'immunity boosters', so here's some information about each to help you decide whether or not you want to give them to your child.

- Omega-3 fatty acids (DHA/EPA): These are important for brain and eye development but, unless your child never eats oily fish or fortified foods, supplements are usually not essential. Algae-based versions are available for plant-based diets.
- Probiotics: There's growing interest in gut health, but research on routine probiotic use in healthy children is still limited. They may help in certain situations (e.g. after antibiotics), but they're not necessary for most children.
- Magnesium: Recently, magnesium supplements, especially in chewable or gummy form, have been marketed to parents with claims of improving sleep, reducing anxiety, or helping with 'restless' behaviour. While magnesium is an important mineral involved in many bodily processes (including muscle and nerve function), most children get enough through their diet, especially if they eat cereals, dairy, leafy greens, or wholegrains. At this stage, there is not enough high-quality evidence to recommend magnesium supplements to aid sleep in young children who are otherwise healthy. If your child is having persistent sleep difficulties, it's better to explore sleep routines, screen time, and potential underlying causes with your GP than to start a supplement without guidance.
- 'Immunity boosters': Many products marketed for children include herbs, high-dose vitamin C, or zinc. These are not generally recommended and may cause side-effects in large amounts.

Can supplements cause harm?

More isn't always better, especially for small bodies:

- Too much vitamin A can affect bone health and liver function. Many over-the-counter multivitamins contain more than young children need.
- Iron can be dangerous in excess. Accidental iron overdoses are a leading cause of poisoning in under-fives, which is why supplements should always be kept out of reach.
- Some gummy supplements contain added sugar and can stick to teeth, increasing the risk of dental decay.

While most supplements are safe when used as directed, it's important to remember that they are not a substitute for a balanced diet. Caring for a young child is full of decisions, and feeding is one of the most emotionally charged. If you've ever worried that your child isn't eating enough greens, you're not alone. Supplements can seem like an easy solution but, in most cases, only a few key nutrients are routinely needed.

In summary, you should:

- focus on food first (variety over perfection)
- give daily vitamin D (plus A and C in the UK) from age one to five
- use multivitamins *only* if recommended by a doctor, pharmacist, or dietitian
- check labels and dosages carefully
- be cautious with social-media advice and always double-check with a professional.

Most importantly, go easy on yourself! Toddlers go through phases; a skipped vegetable here or there is not a crisis. Broccoli might be flavour of the week next week!

DEVELOPMENTAL MILESTONES

The years between two and five are a period of rapid brain growth and development, and healthcare professionals monitor this development by observing your child's developmental milestones. As always, these milestones are a guide for healthcare professionals to flag any possible delays early; they are not a means of judging your child or your parenting skills.

Gross motor skills

Gross motor skills involve the use of large muscle groups that control actions such as walking, running, jumping, and climbing. During the ages of two and five, children become increasingly agile, co-ordinated, and confident in their physical movement.

At age two, many toddlers can walk steadily and begin to run, though they may still fall frequently, and can usually climb on and off furniture. Around this time, children also start to attempt to climb stairs, typically going up by placing both feet on each step and often needing to hold a hand or railing for support.

By age three, children usually gain the co-ordination to walk up stairs using alternate feet, though they may still descend using both feet per step. As balance and strength improve, the ability to confidently go up and down stairs independently becomes more refined. By four and five years old, most children can navigate stairs smoothly (up and down) with alternating feet and without needing to hold on for balance.

Other gross-motor milestones during this stage include kicking and throwing a ball, jumping with both feet, hopping on one foot, riding a tricycle or bike with training wheels, and balancing for several seconds. These activities not only build physical fitness but also promote spatial awareness and confidence.

Supporting gross-motor development means encouraging lots of active play. Offer safe, open spaces and include activities such as climbing playground structures, dancing, playing catch, and, yes, even tackling those stairs (with supervision at first). These daily movements are crucial for developing strength, co-ordination, and independence.

Fine motor skills

While big-body movements capture a lot of attention (and keep you on your toes!), small movements, such as turning pages, using utensils, and holding a crayon, are equally important. Fine-motor development involves strengthening the small muscles of the hands and fingers, which are also closely linked to visual development.

At age two, children begin to stack blocks and scribble with crayons. By age four or five, they can draw shapes, use scissors, dress with minimal help, and even begin writing letters. These skills are fundamental not just for school readiness, but also for self-care and independence.

Encourage development through daily routines by offering your child safe art supplies, involving them in getting dressed, and providing toys that require grasping and manipulation, such as puzzles or building sets.

Around the preschool years, children also refine their visual tracking, hand-eye co-ordination, and depth perception. These are critical for both fine-motor tasks and navigating their environment confidently.

Remember, screentime is not a substitute for real world play, which helps to develop these fine motor skills.

Vision screening and eye health

Between the ages of three and five, most children will be invited for a vision screening appointment with a public-health nurse. This screening checks for strabismus (squint) and refractive errors (such as short- or long-sightedness).

A squint, where one eye may turn inwards, outwards, or upwards, can sometimes be subtle and easily missed by caregivers. If left untreated, it may lead to long-term vision problems. Early detection through routine screening is key, as a squint is most treatable during these early years when the visual system is still developing.

As a parent, you can help by:

- attending scheduled vision screenings when invited
- watching for signs like frequent eye-rubbing, tilting the head to look at things, or noticing if your child seems to bump into objects more than usual
- seeking advice from your doctor or public-health nurse if you notice that your child's eyes appear misaligned
- encouraging daily activities, such as reading picture books, playing with puzzles, or drawing, that support both visual development and fine-motor co-ordination.

Language

'But why?'

You will hear this question more and more in the preschool years, as your child starts to navigate the world using language and reason. This is a time when children absorb language rapidly.

By age two, most children use two-to-three-word phrases, name familiar objects, and understand simple directions. By the age of three, they typically speak in short sentences and ask questions. At four and five, they can tell simple stories, describe events, and hold conversations with both children and adults.

To support this growth, talk to your child throughout the day. Describe what you're doing, ask questions, and read books together. Singing songs, rhyming, and storytelling are also excellent tools to nurture language development.

Common 'sound' challenges

It's completely normal for young children to mispronounce words or substitute sounds as they learn to speak clearly. Some of the most common sound errors in preschool-aged children include:

- substituting 'w' for 'r' (e.g. 'wabbit' for 'rabbit')
- using 't' for 'k' or 'g' (e.g. 'tat' for 'cat')
- dropping final consonants (e.g. 'ca' for 'cat')
- mixing up blends (e.g. 'pane' for 'plane').

These errors are usually part of typical speech development and often resolve naturally by the age of five or six. However, if your child's speech is difficult to understand even to family members by age three or to unfamiliar listeners by age four, it may indicate a need for further evaluation.

While every child develops at their own pace, the following signs may indicate a speech or language delay:

- **By two years:** Says fewer than 50 words, doesn't use two-word phrases (e.g. 'want milk'), and doesn't point to things or respond to simple requests.
- **By three years:** Cannot be understood by parents or caregivers most of the time, limited vocabulary, and doesn't use short sentences or ask questions.
- **By four years:** Speech is unclear to unfamiliar adults, limited use of pronouns or sentence structure, and doesn't engage in pretend play or storytelling.
- **At any age:** Regression or loss of previously acquired speech or language skills.

When and how to seek help

If you notice any red flags or are concerned about your child's communication or language development, trust your instincts and seek guidance early. Here's what you can do:

- Talk to your public-health nurse or GP: They can assess your concerns and refer your child to a speech-and-language therapist if needed.
- Get hearing assessed by an audiologist.
- Don't 'wait and see': Early intervention can significantly improve outcomes, especially before school entry.
- Keep communication flowing at home: Talk often, listen attentively, read books together, and avoid correcting speech errors harshly. Instead, model the correct pronunciation naturally in conversation.

Social and emotional

Social-and-emotional development forms the heart of a child's early relationships and behaviour. It influences how they express emotions, connect with others, and navigate the world around them.

At age two, children often engage in parallel play (playing alongside, rather than with, other children) and may begin to show empathy or defiance. As they approach preschool age, co-operative play emerges, and children start learning to share, take turns, and understand basic rules. By age five, many children can manage their emotions more effectively and can distinguish between reality and make-believe.

You can nurture this area of development by modelling empathy, offering structured choices, maintaining consistent routines, and encouraging peer interaction through playdates or group activities. Emotional validation goes a long way in fostering healthy emotional intelligence.

TOILET TRAINING

One of the biggest milestones your child will reach during these years is toilet training. You might have questions, such as, 'When should I start?', 'What if they're not ready?', 'Why is my toddler suddenly refusing the potty after making great progress?'

The truth is that successful toilet training is less about age and more about readiness. Let's walk through the signs to look for, the common pitfalls to avoid, and some practical tips to make the journey a smooth one.

How to know if your toddler is ready

There's no magic age. Most children are ready somewhere between two and three years, but some are earlier, others later. Signs of readiness include:

- Physical readiness: They can stay dry for at least two hours, or they wake from naps with a dry nappy.
- Awareness: They notice when they are wet or dirty, or they may hide while doing a poo.
- Motor skills: They can walk to the potty or toilet, and they manage some clothing (like pulling trousers up and down).
- Communication: They can tell you (in words, signs, or gestures) that they need to go or that they have just gone.
- Interest: They show curiosity about the toilet or copy what their older siblings and parents do.

If your toddler isn't showing most of these signs, pushing ahead can cause stress for everyone – and may actually delay progress.

Some common pitfalls when it comes to toilet training include:

- Starting too early: Beginning before your child is ready often leads to battles, accidents, and frustration.

- Inconsistency: Switching between full-time training and going back to nappies confuses toddlers.
- Pressure and punishment: Scolding when your child has an accident can cause anxiety and make them withhold wee or poo, leading to constipation.
- Ignoring fears: Some children are frightened of flushing, sitting on a big toilet, or hearing water noises. Dismissing those fears can slow progress.
- Bad timing: Introducing training during a stressful change (new baby, moving house, starting preschool) can backfire.

If your child is ready to start toilet training, here are some practical tips for success:

- Set the stage: Let your toddler watch you or an older sibling use the toilet. Read books or sing songs about potty time.
- Choose the right equipment: A small potty or a child's toilet seat insert plus a step stool can make them feel secure.
- Get the timing right: If your toddler is ready over a holiday period such as Christmas, Easter or summer this may be easier for you logistically.
- Dress for success: Avoid tricky buttons, belts, or tights during training.
- Make it routine: Offer the potty at regular intervals, such as after meals, before bath time, and before bed.
- Celebrate, don't bribe: Praise effort as well as success. Stickers, high fives, or clapping work better than sweets.
- Stay calm about accidents: Treat them matter-of-factly by saying, 'That's okay, let's try again.'
- Night training comes later: Many children are dry in the day before they are dry at night – this is normal.

If you're worried about persistent constipation, pain, or regression after weeks of progress, talk to your GP or public-health nurse for guidance. You can find more information on constipation and diarrhoea in Chapter 8, from page 204.

Toilet training is not a race, and comparing your child to others will only create pressure. Look for readiness cues, be patient, and keep the tone positive. Remember – every child gets there in their own time.

TANTRUMS, MELTDOWNS, AND OPPOSITION

Around this age, your child might start to grapple with big emotions.

You have no doubt heard of the 'terrible twos' and 'threenagers'. Certainly, this age cohort can get a bit sassy as they try to exert some independence, but it is possible to navigate behavioural bumps with compassion – for your child and for yourself.

Honestly, there is no telling what might trigger a tantrum in a toddler. One that we still laugh about in my house is the 'Great Jelly Disaster', when my then three-year-old was served jelly for dessert and could not cope with the fact that it did not retain the exact shape of the jelly mould when it was placed in her bowl. It made no sense to anyone why this would be so upsetting, but no doubt she had her reasons in her little toddler mind.

Understanding what drives behaviours like tantrums and meltdowns can help you respond in a calm and constructive way, while still setting healthy boundaries.

Why do tantrums happen?

Tantrums occur when a child feels overwhelmed – physically, emotionally, or cognitively. This may be due to:

- frustration with limited language or motor skills
- fatigue, hunger, overstimulation, or changes in routine

- difficulty in handling transitions or not getting their way
- desire for independence, clashing with limits set by adults.

Meltdowns versus tantrums: is there a difference?

While tantrums can be partly voluntary and may stop when the child gets what they want, meltdowns are typically a full emotional overload, often seen in tired, overwhelmed, or neurodivergent children (e.g. those with sensory sensitivities or autism).

A meltdown is not manipulative or deliberate; it is a sign that a child has lost the ability to self-regulate and needs support, not punishment. If your child is experiencing a meltdown, remembering the following will help you to respond calmly and effectively.

- Stay calm and grounded: Your calm presence helps co-regulate your child's emotions. Use a soft, steady voice and keep your body language neutral, even when their behaviour is explosive.
- Validate the feeling, not the behaviour: Say things like, 'I can see you're really upset' or 'It's okay to feel angry, but not okay to hit.' Naming emotions helps children begin to understand and manage them over time.
- Set clear, consistent boundaries: Children need limits to feel safe. Keep rules simple and consistent. For example, 'I won't let you throw things. Let's take a break and calm down.' Follow through with kindness, not threats.
- Use redirection and choices: Offer two acceptable options to give your child a sense of control. For example, 'You can wear your red shoes or your blue ones.' This helps prevent power struggles before they escalate.
- Teach emotional regulation in calm moments: After the storm has passed, gently talk about what happened.

Introduce simple coping tools, such as deep breaths, counting to five, or using a 'calm corner'. Storybooks about emotions can be great teaching tools.

Don't forget to be kind to yourself. These big emotions our toddlers experience can provoke pretty strong emotions in us as well. You might need a bit of time to yourself after a particularly emotional day. You might feel bad after expressing frustration to your child or feel you could have handled things better. But don't forget, for every one time that things have been frustrating or fraught, there have been ten times that you absolutely aced it with your toddler.

When to seek support

Some emotional outbursts are more frequent or intense than expected for certain ages. You may want to consult your GP, public-health nurse, or a child psychologist if:

- tantrums are violent, very frequent, or regularly last longer than 15–20 minutes
- your child hurts themselves or others
- there's a regression in other areas of development (e.g. speech, toilet training, play)
- your child has persistent difficulties with transitions or sensory input.

Early support can help you and your child build better communication, emotional resilience, and coping strategies, especially if there's an underlying developmental or sensory issue.

There's a lot going on between the ages of two and five regarding developmental milestones, so here's a handy summary of what healthcare professionals look out for.

Age	Gross Motor	Fine Motor and Vision	Communication	Social and Emotional
Two years	• Walks and runs steadily • walks upstairs with support, both feet per step	• Stacks 4–6 blocks, scribbles • tracks moving objects visually	• Uses 2–3-word phrases • may mispronounce sounds • red flag if fewer than 50 words or not combining words	• Parallel play • shows defiance
Three years	• Climbs stairs with alternating feet • walks downstairs with both feet per step	• Turns book pages, draws a circle • public-health vision screening begins in many areas	• Speaks in short sentences • asks questions • red flag if not understood by family	• Imitates adults • shows affection
Four years	• Walks up and down stairs confidently using alternating feet without support	• Cuts with scissors, draws basic shapes • watch for signs of squint or vision problems	• Tells stories, knows colours • some unclear sounds normal • red flag if speech is unclear to strangers	• Plays co-operatively • understands rules
Five years	• Skips, runs with agility, climbs and descends stairs fluidly without help	• Writes some letters, ties shoelaces • visual skills well developed for classroom readiness	• Speaks clearly in full sentences • may still struggle with 'r', 'th' sounds • red flag if significant clarity issues persist	• Follows rules • distinguishes real from make-believe

SLEEP

Between the ages of two and five, children undergo many changes in how they sleep, transitioning from toddler to preschooler and, sometimes, bringing sleep struggles along the way. As a paediatrician, I'm often asked about nap routines, night terrors, snoring, and bedwetting.

How much sleep?

Children between two and five years old typically need 11–13 hours of sleep in a 24-hour period. This may include a nap for younger children but, by age five, most no longer nap during the day.

- Ages 2–3: One afternoon nap (about 1–2 hours) is common and still needed by most children.
- Age 4: Some children begin to drop the nap or skip it occasionally.
- Age 5: Most are ready to go without a nap but benefit from some quiet time in the afternoon.

Watch for signs of tiredness and let that guide whether a nap is still appropriate.

When to drop the nap

Naps don't stop all at once. Your child may go back and forth for a while. Here are signs they're ready:

- They take a long time to fall asleep at bedtime after napping.
- They start waking earlier in the morning.
- They cope well without a nap and aren't cranky or overtired.

If your child seems to be dropping their nap, try offering a quiet time instead – a break with books, music, or toys in a calm space. It still provides rest without pushing sleep.

Moving from a cot to a bed

Moving from a cot to a bed is a major step in your child's development. It usually happens between 18 months and 3.5 years, depending on your child's readiness and safety. There's no rush, but if your child starts climbing out of their cot, appears cramped, or you're expecting a new baby, it might be time to make the move.

When it comes to beds, many parents ask whether they should go straight to a single bed or opt for a toddler bed as a stepping stone. The pros of a toddler bed are that it is lower to the ground, may have inbuilt side rails, and it feels less intimidating than a full-sized bed. The cons are that it may be outgrown quickly, and you will then have the cost of upgrading to a full-sized bed. Some families skip the toddler bed entirely and go straight to a low single bed, especially if they're keen to invest in a bed that will last several years. Others prefer the toddler bed. There's no right or wrong. It's about what works for your child, your space, and your budget.

Here are some tips for a smooth transition from cot to bed (regardless of bed type):

- Involve your child: Let them choose bedding or help 'set up' the new bed.
- Keep the routine consistent: Keep bath, books, and bedtime the same to maintain familiarity.
- Consider a bed guard or push the bed against a wall to prevent falls (especially if skipping the toddler bed).
- Expect some trial and error: Many children test boundaries when they're no longer physically contained. Calm, consistent returns to bed help reinforce limits.

Sleep challenges

Your friend's child might be sleeping blissfully through the night by now while you are still being woken up by your toddler. Why is this happening? Well, firstly, do not feel bad about it. There might be a few simple fixes, or your child might have an underlying problem that needs medical review. Some common sleep challenges faced by children aged two to five are bedtime resistance, night wakings, and overtiredness.

Sometimes, your little one is just having too much fun to spoil it all by going to bed. When you encounter resistance like this, remember they are little creatures of routine. A predictable routine in the hour leading up to bedtime will help to get your toddler or preschooler mentally prepared. That might be something like a favourite cartoon, a bath and then a story – or another routine that fits into your family life.

Waking at night is still very common in this age group. Make sure the sleep environment is cool, quiet, and dark. Blackout curtains or blinds can be a big help during the long summer evenings.

Overtiredness actually keeps kids awake or causes them to wake during the night. I could always tell when my younger child was overtired. She would conk out as soon as her head hit the pillow and be wide awake again at 11 pm. Keeping bedtimes regular is important in this age group, and they should generally be in bed by 7–8 pm.

Sometimes, your little one might wake because of a night terror or nightmare. Night terrors often occur in the first half of the night. Your child may cry out, appear frightened, and not respond, but they're not fully awake and won't remember it.

Nightmares happen later in the night (during lighter sleep). Your child may wake up scared and seek comfort, often remembering the dream.

- For night terrors: Let it pass. Don't wake your child, just ensure they're safe.
- For nightmares: Offer calm reassurance. A nightlight or bedtime chat can help reduce fears.

Both are usually normal but, if episodes are frequent, worsening, or disrupting daily life, speak to your GP.

Snoring and sleep apnoea

Some parents tell me that their toddler or preschooler seems tired all the time, despite going to bed early and getting 10–12 hours' sleep. When I hear this, I ask two questions: do they wake up refreshed or seem tired, and do they snore?

Occasional snoring during a cold is normal, but regular or loud snoring can be a red flag.

Signs of possible obstructive sleep apnoea:

- loud snoring most nights
- pauses in breathing or gasping in sleep
- restless sleep, bedwetting, or sleeping in strange positions (e.g. neck extended)
- daytime tiredness or hyperactivity.

Obstructive sleep apnoea is often caused by enlarged tonsils or adenoids, so it's important to raise concerns with your GP. They may refer your child for a sleep study or to an ENT (ear, nose, and throat) specialist. Treatment may involve monitoring, surgery (such as a tonsillectomy), or other interventions depending on the severity of your child's condition.

Bedwetting

Bedwetting (nocturnal enuresis) is very common in toddlers and preschoolers and is rarely a sign of a kidney or bladder problem.

It is usually due to the bladder still developing or the child sleeping deeply.

What's normal:

- wetting the bed a few times a week up to age seven
- no other signs of illness or stress
- dry during the day.

See your GP if:

- bedwetting continues past age seven
- your child was dry for several months and starts wetting the bed again
- there's pain when urinating or day-time accidents.

You can support your child when they wet the bed by doing the following:

- Avoid blame or punishment.
- Encourage them to use the toilet before bed.
- Use waterproof sheets or bed pads.
- Limit fluids in the hour before sleep (but don't restrict drinks during the day).

Bedwetting is common up to the age of seven, and even children who have been dry at night for a spell may have the occasional 'accident'. I always had clean sheets to hand for middle-of-the-night changes until my kids had been dry at night for about six months.

ILLNESSES AND ACCIDENTS

Your little one will continue to get several viral infections per year, usually concentrated in the winter months. As they grow and their immune system matures, they will be better able to cope with illness.

Whilst viral illness causing symptoms of the common cold are frequent in this age group, some toddlers may develop recurring ear infections, tonsillitis, or urinary tract infections (UTIs).

Ear infections

Ear infections are one of the most common childhood illnesses, especially in babies and toddlers. While most are mild and resolve on their own, some require medical attention and treatment.

An ear infection (called 'otitis media') is an inflammation of the middle ear (the space behind the eardrum) usually caused by a viral or bacterial infection. It often follows a cold, when mucus and fluid build up in the ear and create the perfect environment for germs to grow.

Babies and toddlers can't always express what they're feeling, so recognising the common symptoms of an ear infection is key:

- irritability or increased crying
- fever (over 38°C)
- pulling or tugging at the ear
- poor sleep
- loss of appetite or trouble feeding (sucking can cause increased ear pressure)
- fluid or pus draining from the ear
- difficulty hearing or not responding to sounds
- older children might complain of a pain in their ear.

Sometimes, the only sign may be disrupted sleep or general discomfort.

Treatment for ear infections

Most ear infections, especially those caused by viruses, will clear up on their own within a couple of days. For many children, watchful waiting is all that's needed.

You can help keep your child comfortable by:

- giving them infant paracetamol or ibuprofen, as advised for their age
- giving them plenty of fluids and cuddles
- keeping their head slightly raised when resting (this helps fluid to drain out of the Eustachian tubes into the back of the throat).

Antibiotics are only prescribed in certain circumstances, and most ear infections don't benefit from them. There are times, however, when they are the right call. If your child is still showing signs of discomfort for more than one day despite regular pain relief, consult your GP, who may recommend antibiotics if they identify any of the following issues:

- your child is under six months old
- the infection is in both ears
- there's fluid or pus leaking from the ear
- they're particularly unwell, with a high fever or ongoing pain
- they've had recurrent infections.

If antibiotics are prescribed, it's important to finish the full course, even if your child seems better halfway through.

Ear infections can temporarily affect your child's hearing. Fluid in the middle ear (even after the infection has gone) can cause muffled hearing for weeks. This condition is known as 'glue ear'. It often resolves by itself, but if it lingers for more than three months or if you notice your child falling behind with speech or struggling in noisy environments, it's worth getting their hearing tested.

Grommets

If your child has ongoing issues with fluid in the ears or frequent infections, an ENT (ears, nose, and throat) specialist may suggest grommets. These are tiny plastic tubes that are inserted into the eardrum during a short operation (usually under general anaesthetic). They help air circulate and prevent fluid build-up. Your child might be considered for grommets if:

- they've had three or more ear infections in six months
- they've had persistent glue ear for over three months with signs of hearing loss or speech delay.

The procedure is quick and many parents report a big improvement in their child's hearing and language development.

While most ear infections are harmless, some symptoms may indicate a more serious issue. Get urgent medical help from your GP or emergency department if your child has any of the following:

- has a very high fever (over 39°C) or seems floppy or unusually drowsy
- has a stiff neck, sensitivity to light, or a severe headache
- has swelling or redness behind the ear, or the ear looks like it's sticking out
- develops vomiting, fits (seizures), or confusion
- has fluid or blood coming from the ear after a head injury.

These signs could suggest complications such as mastoiditis (a bacterial infection of the bone behind the ear) or other infections that need immediate care.

Tonsillitis

Tonsillitis, that nasty inflammation of the tonsils, is a familiar visitor to many homes with young children. If it keeps coming back or starts affecting sleep, it may be time to consider whether your child needs their tonsils removed.

Tonsillitis is an infection of the tonsils, which are the two soft lumps at the back of the throat. The tonsils are part of the immune system, acting as the body's early-warning system for incoming germs. It's a bit ironic that they are so often the first to get infected!

In toddlers, tonsillitis is most commonly caused by viruses, though sometimes bacteria like Streptococcus (strep throat) are to blame.

Symptoms to watch out for include:

- a sore throat, though your toddler might just be fussy or refuse food
- a fever (38°C or more)
- bad breath
- snoring or noisy breathing
- swollen lymph nodes in the neck
- white spots on the tonsils.

Most cases of tonsillitis are viral and won't respond to antibiotics but, if your GP suspects a bacterial infection, particularly strep throat, they may prescribe them. These can help shorten the illness and reduce complications. However, if it is a viral infection, antibiotics won't help. It's important to remember that overuse of antibiotics can contribute to resistance and can have side-effects (tummy upset, rashes, and yeast infections).

The 'wait and see' approach is often best, unless your child is particularly unwell, the symptoms are severe, or there's a confirmed bacterial cause. See Chapter 15, page 363, for more information on tonsilitis.

Tonsillitis can usually be managed at home, but seek medical help if:

- your child is drooling and struggling to swallow or breathe
- there is neck stiffness, a very high fever (39°C or more), severe pain, or a fever that does not respond to treatment with paracetamol or ibuprofen
- your child is lethargic, pale, or difficult to wake
- you see blood in your child's saliva or vomit.

These symptoms could indicate a more serious complication, such as a peritonsillar abscess or airway obstruction, and will require prompt assessment.

Do the tonsils need to come out?

No parent wants to jump straight to surgery and, thankfully, in most cases, it's not necessary. But for some toddlers, a tonsillectomy (removal of the tonsils) can be life-changing.

It might be considered if your child:

- has seven or more episodes of tonsillitis in one year
- has five episodes per year over two consecutive years
- has significant obstructive sleep apnoea due to large tonsils
- has difficulty swallowing
- is frequently absent from crèche/nursery due to illness.

Modern tonsillectomy is a safe procedure but, like all surgeries, it's not without risks. These include:

- bleeding (especially 5–10 days post-op – watch for spitting or vomiting blood)

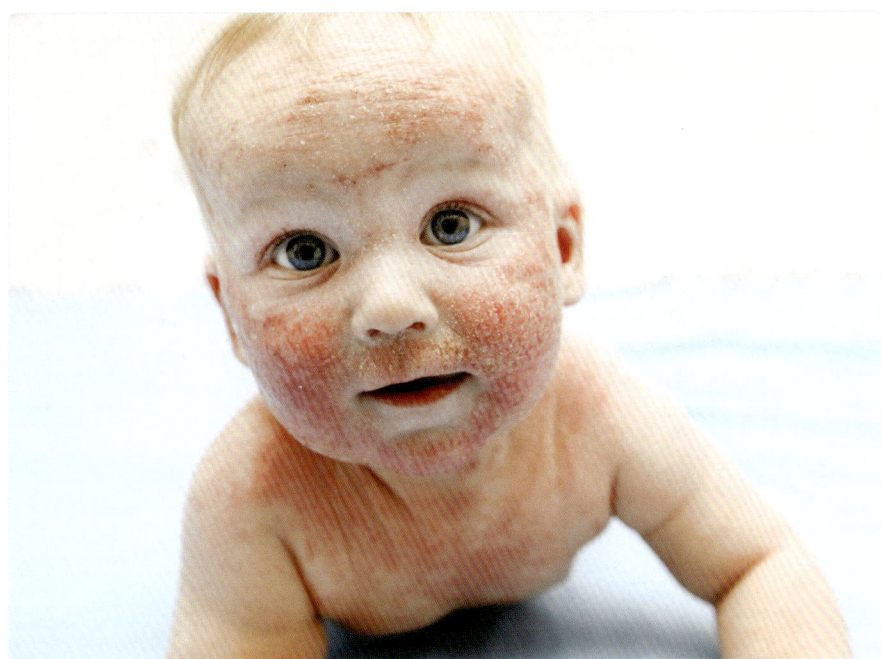

In babies under six months, **eczema** typically appears on the cheeks, forehead, and scalp, although it can also appear on the arms, legs, or torso. The skin may look red, rough, and scaly, or it may even be oozing in more severe cases.

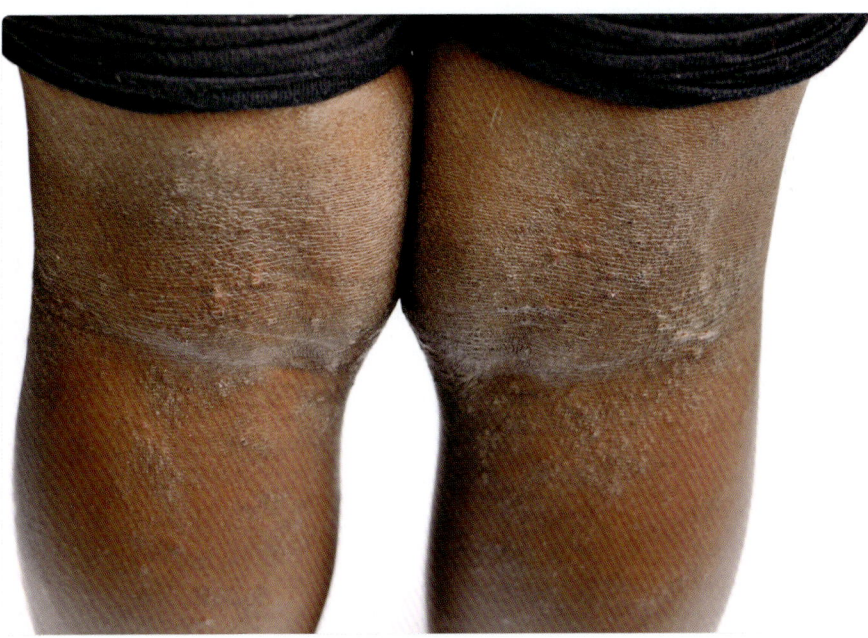

Eczema is common in children with a family history of allergies, asthma, or hay fever. Children with this condition are more prone to skin infections because of the disrupted skin barrier.

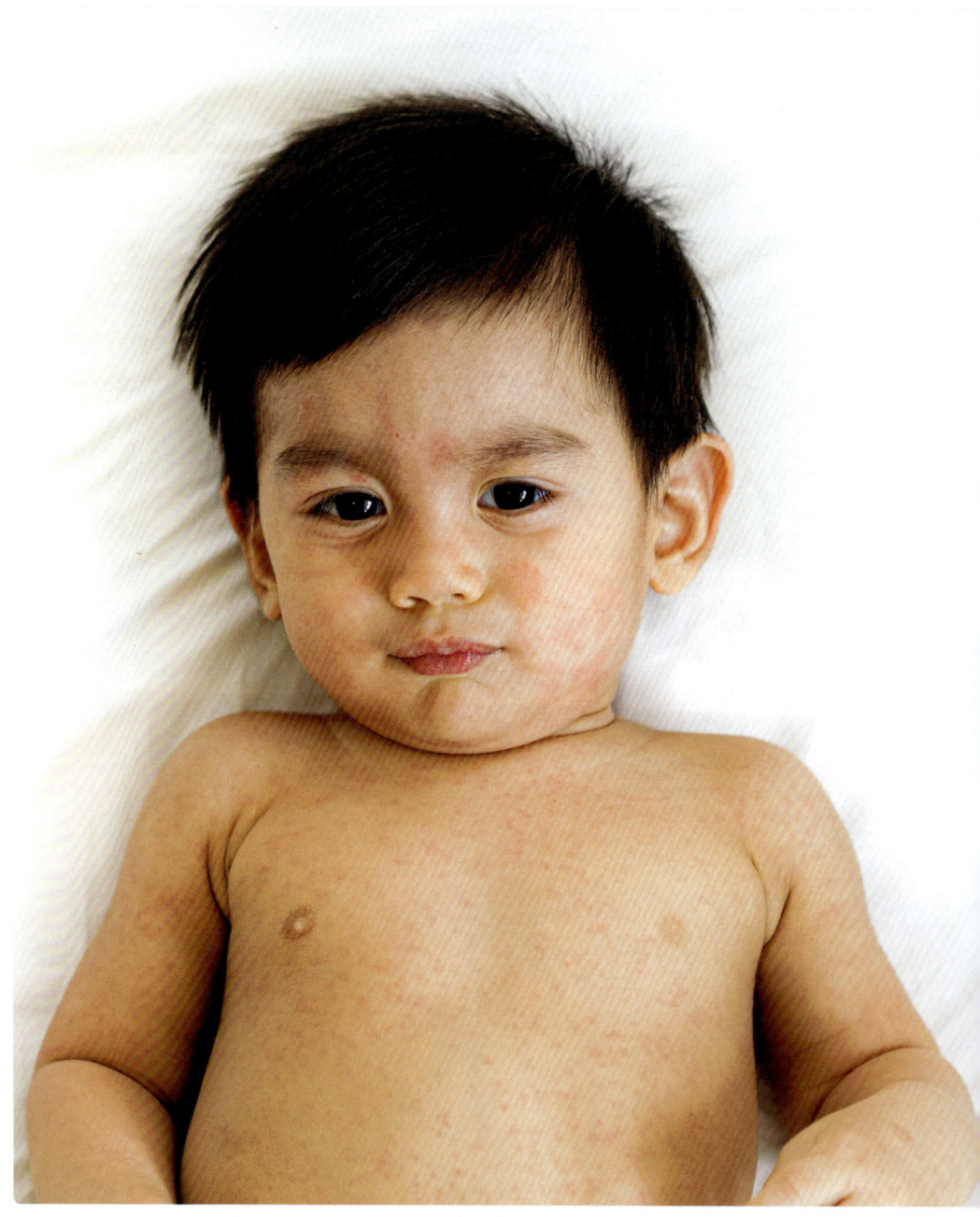

Roseola is a common viral infection. Children usually have a fever for three to six days, followed by a pink, bumpy rash that starts on the torso, then spreads to the face and limbs. The rash is not itchy and lasts for about two days.

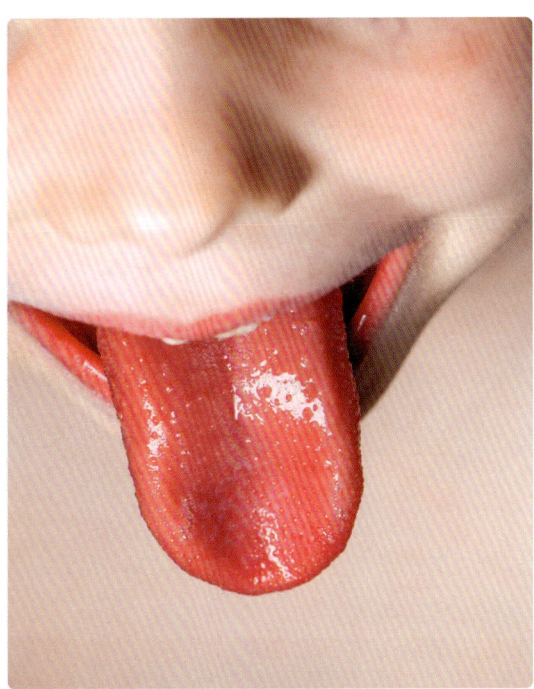

One of the symptoms of **scarlet fever** is 'strawberry tongue' where the tongue is bumpy and bright red. Other symptoms include sore throat, fever, and a fine, sandpaper-like rash starting on the chest.

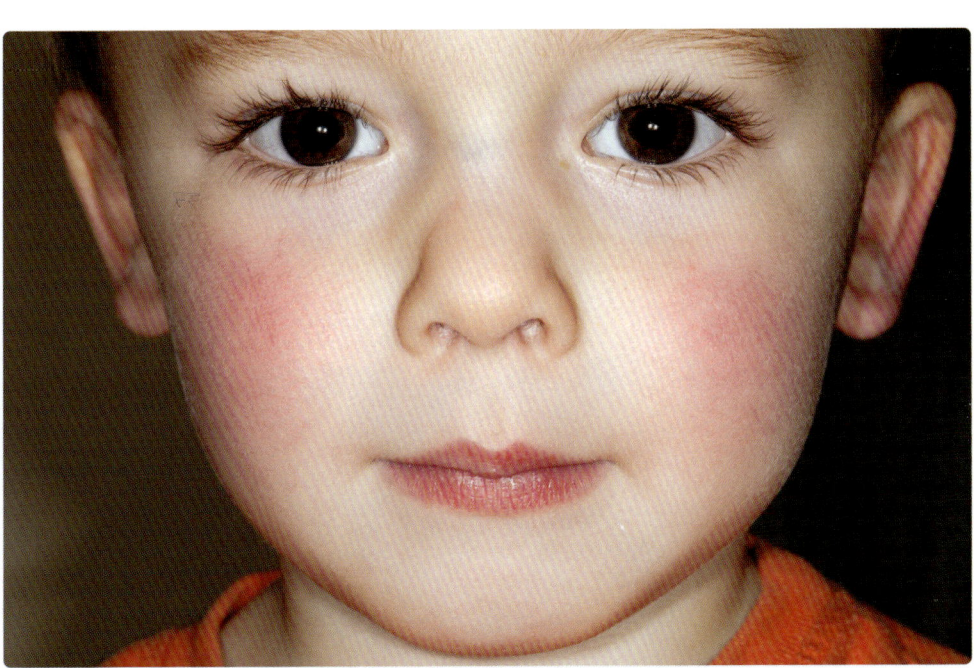

Red, flushed cheeks are a hallmark sign of **slapped cheek disease**. The rash may later spread to the body in a light, lacy pattern. Caused by parvovirus B19, this viral rash is usually mild in children.

Cold sores on the lip are commonly caused by **herpes simplex** virus type 1 (HSV-1). After the first infection, the virus can remain dormant and occasionally reactivate, causing similar small blisters. In some cases, HSV-1 can lead to complications such as painful mouth ulcers (herpetic stomatitis) so monitoring symptoms is important. Children with eczema may develop a serious complication called eczema herpeticum.

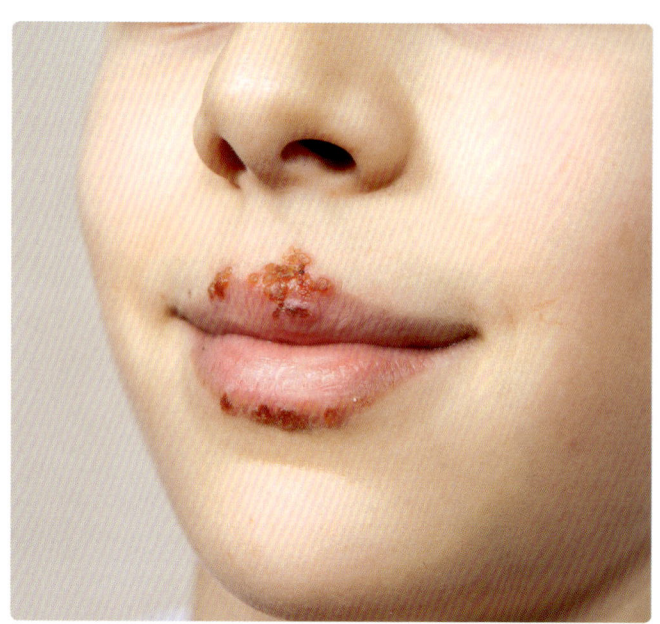

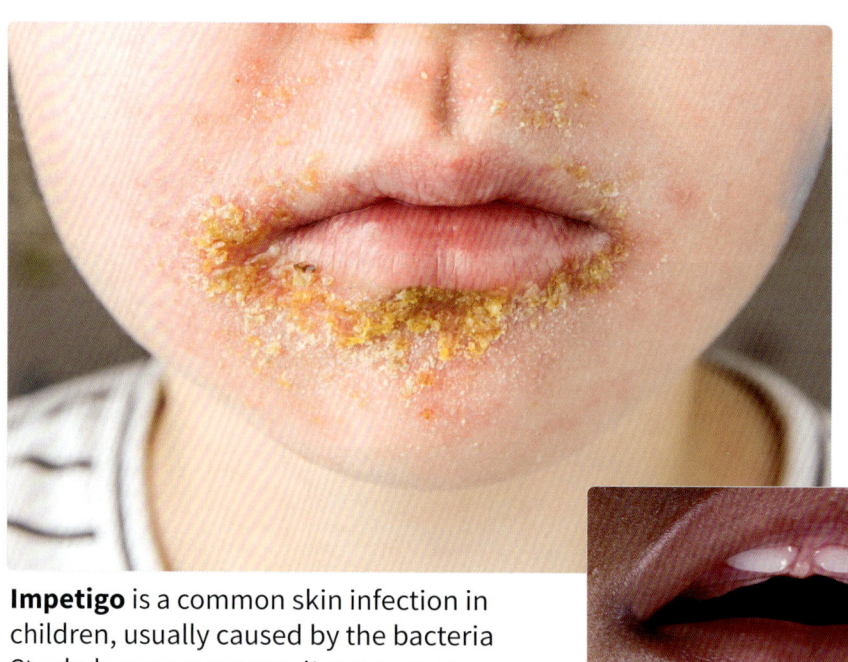

Impetigo is a common skin infection in children, usually caused by the bacteria Staphylococcus aureus. It appears as small blisters or honey-coloured crusts and spreads easily through close contact.

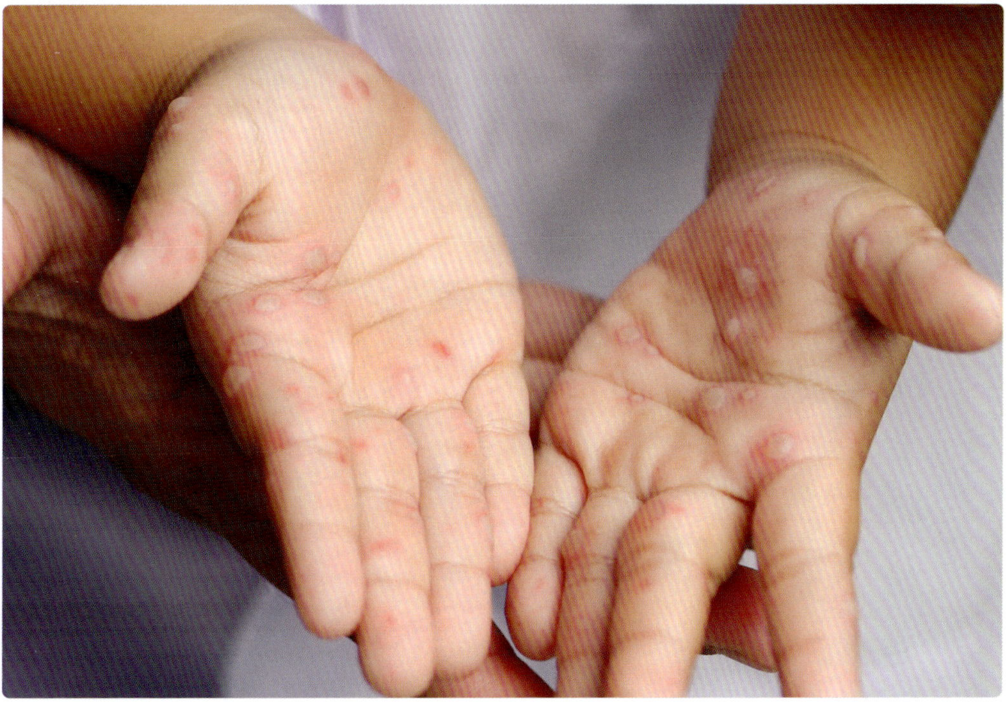

Hand, foot, and mouth disease is caused most often by coxsackieviruses, leading to small blisters on the hands, feet, bottom, and inside the mouth. It is usually mild but can cause discomfort from mouth sores and fever. Dehydration may occur because eating and drinking can be painful.

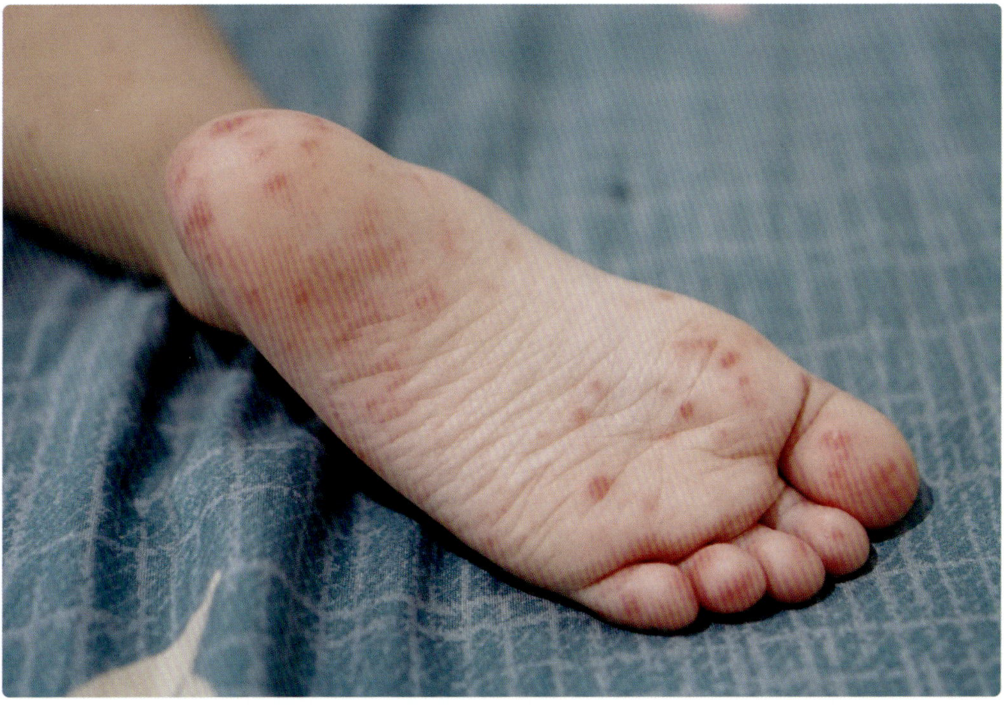

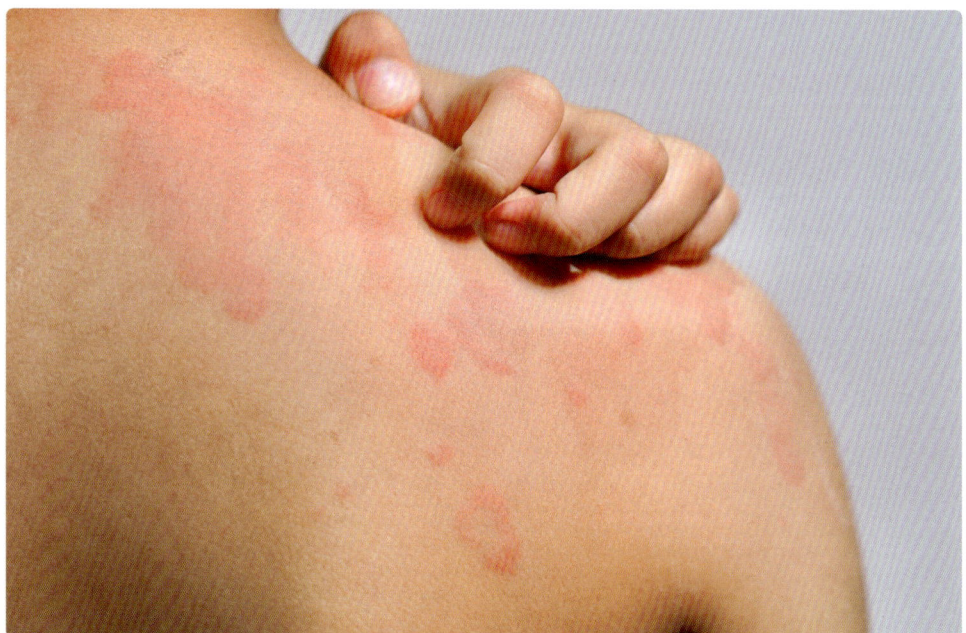

Urticaria, or hives, appears as raised, itchy welts on the skin and is usually caused by an allergic reaction, infection, or other triggers. On darker skin, the welts may appear darker than the surrounding skin rather than red, but are still raised and itchy. Most cases are temporary, but persistent or widespread hives should be assessed by a healthcare professional.

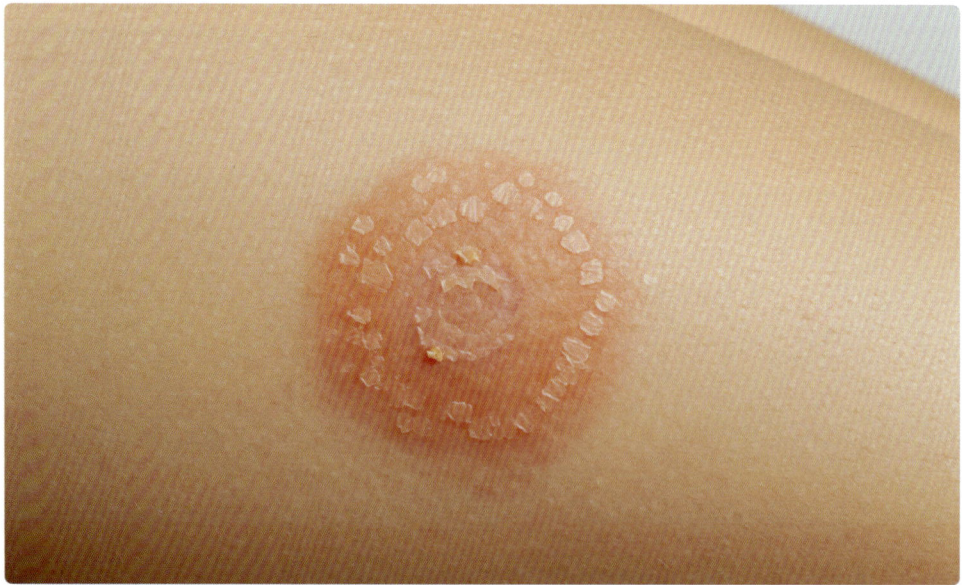

Ringworm is a common fungal infection and appears as a circular, scaly rash. When it affects the scalp it is called tinea capitis, which often shows as patchy hair loss, scaling, or small black dots where hairs have broken off. On dark skin, ringworm may look less red and more like a slightly darker or lighter ring with a subtle scaling around the edges.

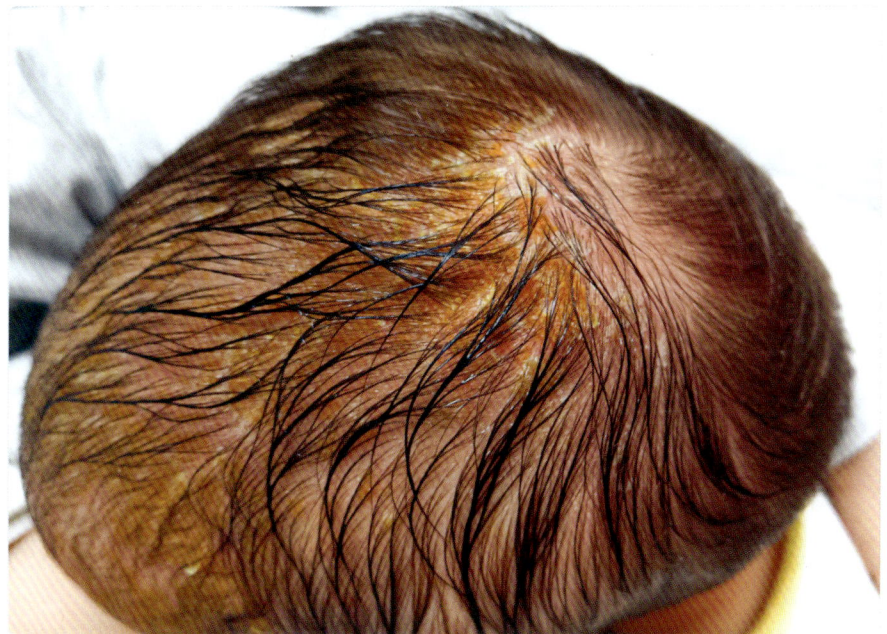

Cradle cap is a harmless skin condition caused by the build-up of dry skin and natural oils on your baby's scalp. The main symptom is patches of greasy, scaly skin, mainly on the scalp, but it can be present on the eyebrows and even in the nappy area.

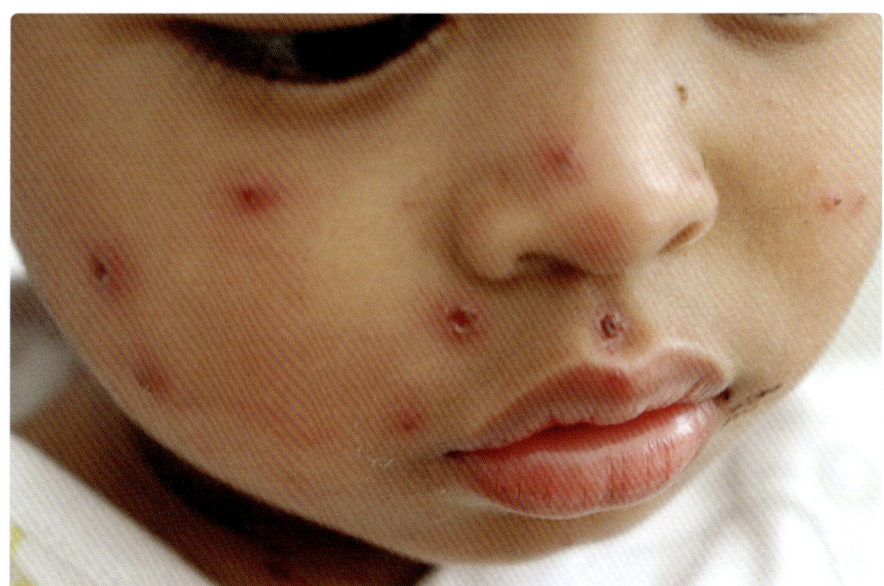

Chickenpox is caused by the varicella-zoster virus and produces an itchy rash with spots that turn into fluid-filled blisters before crusting over. Children may also have fever and tiredness during the illness. While usually mild, chickenpox can sometimes lead to complications such as skin infection.

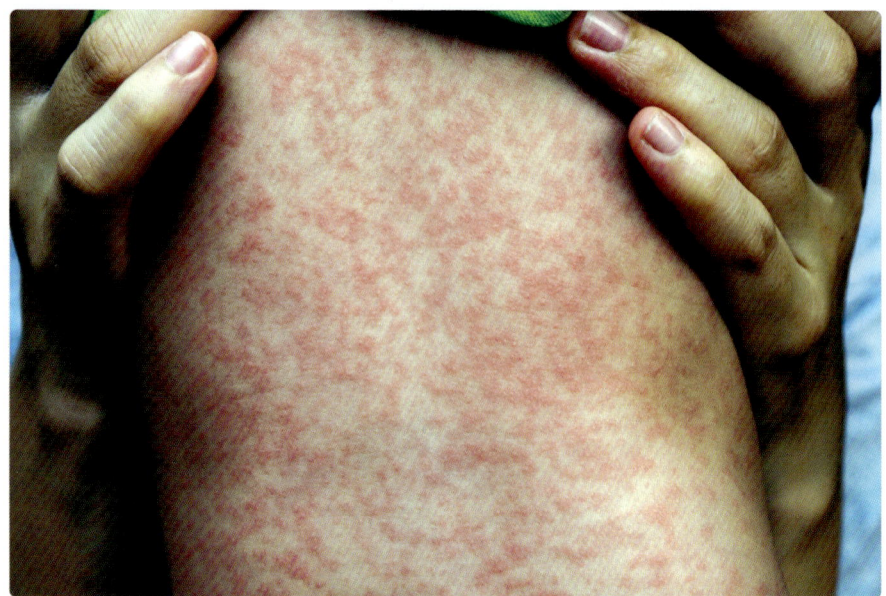

Measles is caused by the measles virus and produces a blotchy red rash that typically spreads from the head downward. Other signs include high fever, cough, runny nose, red eyes, and tiny white 'Koplik spots' inside the cheeks. Measles can lead to serious complications such as ear infections, pneumonia, or, rarely, inflammation of the brain. Vaccination protects children from measles infection.

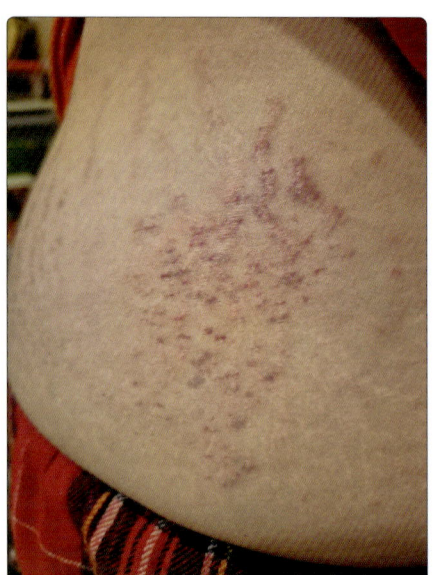 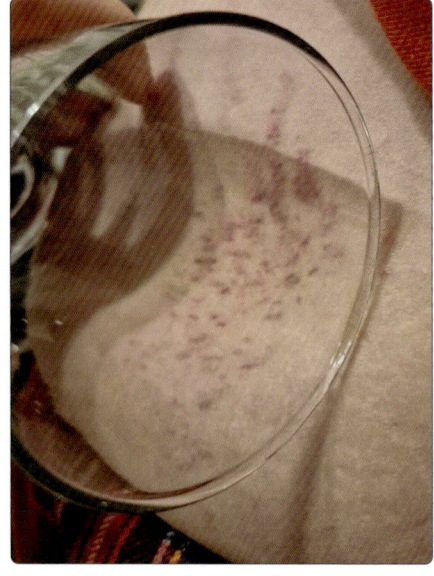

A **non-blanching rash** can be a sign of serious illness, such as sepsis or meningitis. You can check if a rash is non-blanching by pressing a clear tumbler over the rash. If it does not fade under the pressure of the glass, it is a non blanching rash.

- pain (can last 1–2 weeks)
- infection
- dehydration (toddlers may refuse to drink due to throat pain).

It's also worth noting that tonsils sometimes shrink over time, so watchful waiting may be advised.

Wheeze

When my kids were small, the winter brought a cacophony of coughing and wheezing. Every virus that came our way seemed to, as my granny used to say, 'go to their chest'. One of my children was later diagnosed with asthma, but recurring wheeze in a toddler or preschooler does not always lead to a diagnosis of asthma.

Let's take a closer look at recurrent viral wheeze versus asthma, and what you need to know.

What is recurrent viral wheeze?
Recurrent viral wheeze is common in children between ages two and five. It often occurs in response to viral infections, such as colds or flu, and may cause:

- wheezing or whistling sounds when breathing
- coughing
- mild shortness of breath.

The key here is that the wheeze usually appears only during viral infections and children are typically well between illnesses.

What is asthma in young children?
Asthma is a chronic condition where the airways are inflamed and more sensitive, making them narrow more easily. Children with asthma may wheeze or cough even without a cold, and symptoms can be triggered by:

- allergies
- exercise
- irritants (like cigarette smoke).

Asthma can also cause more persistent symptoms, such as nighttime coughing or repeated breathing difficulties. Sometimes children with asthma do not have an obvious wheeze and persistent nighttime coughing is their main symptom.

Recurrent viral wheeze v asthma

Feature	Recurrent Viral Wheeze	Asthma
When wheeze occurs	Mostly during colds	Can occur anytime
Between episodes	Usually well	May have ongoing symptoms
Triggers	Viral infections	Allergens, exercise, irritants, infections
Long-term risk	Often improves by school age	May continue into later childhood or adulthood

Treatments: are they different?

When it comes to recurrent viral wheeze, the approach is often supportive. Most children improve with simple care at home, keeping them comfortable, making sure they stay well hydrated, and closely watching their breathing. If a wheezing episode becomes more noticeable, a paediatrician might suggest a short course of a 'rescue' inhaler, like salbutamol, which helps open the airways temporarily. Generally, these children do not need daily medication, since their symptoms tend to flare only with viral infections.

Asthma, on the other hand, usually requires a more structured plan. Children with asthma often benefit from daily inhaled medicines that reduce inflammation in their airways, helping prevent flare-ups before they start. Even with these medications, there's usually a rescue inhaler prescribed for sudden symptoms. Families are encouraged to work with their paediatrician to create an individual asthma action plan, which explains exactly what to do if symptoms worsen and how to respond in emergencies. This plan gives parents clear steps to manage their child's breathing with confidence.

In both situations, parents play a key role in observing patterns, noting triggers, and creating a supportive environment. Reducing exposure to smoke or strong irritants can help prevent episodes, whether it's viral wheeze or asthma.

Many young children experience wheezing, and it can be frightening. The good news is that recurrent viral wheeze is common and often outgrown, while asthma is manageable with the right treatment plan.

(See A–Z chapter, page 305 for more information on breathing problems in children.)

Urinary tract infections (UTIs)

UTIs can be hard to detect, because they are not obvious and, as parents, we don't think of them straightaway. Both of my girls had UTIs as toddlers. You'd think after going through it with my first, I would have been on the ball for my second, but no – I was just as baffled the second time round when my three-year-old started to complain of tummy pain, cried when she peed, and spiked a fever.

A UTI occurs when bacteria, usually Escherichia coli (E. coli, commonly found in poo), enter the urinary tract – that's the bladder, kidneys, ureters, or urethra. In toddlers, this often happens when bacteria from the skin or bottom spread into the urethra. The urethra is the tube that carries urine out of the bladder and into the toilet (or potty or nappy!). Bacteria can travel up this tube and into the bladder, causing pain and irritation.

Factors that increase the risk of a UTI include:

- infrequent urination or holding in pee for too long
- incomplete bladder emptying

- constipation (we'll talk more about this in Chapter 8)
- poor toilet hygiene or improper wiping
- anatomical issues, which are thankfully rare.

In this age group, UTIs are more common in girls than boys because that little tube (the urethra) that goes from the bladder to the outside is shorter in girls than in boys. However, UTIs can still happen in boys.

UTIs can be sneaky in toddlers, so some of the signs to watch out for include:

- fever (38°C or more) with no obvious source
- crying or discomfort when passing urine
- foul-smelling, cloudy, or bloody urine
- frequent urination or accidents
- tummy pain, vomiting, or refusal to eat
- irritability or just seeming 'off'.

If your child has a fever and no clear reason (like a cold or ear infection), it's always worth checking a urine sample. This is something both GPs and hospital paediatric teams do routinely.

When a UTI is suspected, a urine sample will be taken, usually via a urine bag, clean-catch sample, or catheter if needed in very young children. If a UTI is confirmed, the treatment involves:

- antibiotics, either liquid or tablets, for about three to seven days depending on the child's age and the severity of the infection
- fluids and pain relief (such as paracetamol or ibuprofen)
- a stay in hospital for intravenous antibiotics if your child is vomiting or very unwell.

Remember, it's vital to complete the full course of antibiotics, even if your child seems better after a few days, to ensure the infection is properly cleared.

In cases of recurrent UTIs, your GP may refer your child for ultrasound or other tests to check their kidneys and bladder. These tests are usually straightforward and help identify any underlying problems.

How to prevent UTIs
Good hygiene can help prevent infections. Wipe girls front to back to avoid transferring bacteria to the urethra.

For boys, clean the penis gently during baths, no special soaps or scrubbing are needed. It does not help to retract the foreskin – forcibly pulling it back can cause pain, damage, and even infections. It's enough to wash the outside gently. The foreskin will naturally start to retract in its own time, often after age five, sometimes later. Routine circumcision is not recommended for the prevention of UTIs, though it may be considered in boys with recurrent UTIs and infections of the foreskin.

Managing constipation (see page 204) is also very important in helping to prevent UTIs, as the two often go hand in hand. But why is this? A backed-up bowel can press against the bladder, preventing it from emptying properly and enabling bacteria to grow.

Watch out for hard stools, pain when your child passes stools, or a toddler who goes days without pooping. Ensuring a diet rich in fibre, hydration, and regular toilet time helps to keep everything moving and reduces the risk of infections.

Circumcision

While circumcision is not routinely performed in Ireland, there are some medical reasons why a doctor might recommend it. Most boys will not require this procedure, as the foreskin develops naturally and can be cared for safely with gentle hygiene. By understanding foreskin development and keeping an eye out for any warning signs, parents can ensure their child's genital health and make informed decisions if a doctor recommends circumcision. Regardless of whether circumcision is performed for medical or for religious or cultural reasons, it should only be done by a trained and registered surgeon in a clinical setting.

What is circumcision?

Circumcision is a surgical procedure that removes the foreskin, the fold of skin that covers the tip of the penis.

How the foreskin develops

At birth, a baby boy's foreskin is naturally fused to the glans (the tip of the penis) and cannot be fully retracted. This is completely normal. Over time, usually by age 3 to 5, the foreskin gradually loosens and becomes retractable. Full retraction may not occur until adolescence. The foreskin serves an important role in protecting the sensitive tip of the penis from infection and injury during these early years.

Medical reasons for circumcision

Doctors may recommend circumcision in the following situations:

- Phimosis: This occurs when the foreskin is too tight to be pulled back over the tip of the penis. While mild cases often resolve naturally with age, severe cases can cause pain, urinary problems, or recurrent infections.
- Recurrent infections: Some boys experience repeated infections under the foreskin (balanitis) or urinary tract infections (UTIs) that do not improve with other treatments. Circumcision can reduce the risk of these infections.
- Paraphimosis: This is a rare but urgent condition where a tight foreskin gets stuck behind the glans and cannot return to its normal position. Circumcision may be necessary to prevent complications.
- Other medical conditions: In rare cases, circumcision may be advised for conditions such as congenital abnormalities of the penis or certain dermatological issues affecting the foreskin.

Caring for the foreskin

Good foreskin care can prevent some of the problems that might lead to circumcision. Here's what parents need to know:

- Do not force retraction: Never pull back a baby's foreskin forcibly. It will separate naturally over time.
- Gentle cleaning: Once the foreskin becomes retractable, gently pull it back and wash the area with warm water. Soap is generally not needed, as it can irritate sensitive skin.
- Dry thoroughly: After washing, gently dry the area to prevent moisture-related irritation or infections.
- Observe for symptoms: Redness, swelling, discharge, or pain are signs to consult your GP.

When to Seek Medical Advice

Contact your GP if your child has:

- painful urination or difficulty urinating
- swelling or redness at the tip of the penis
- recurring infections under the foreskin
- any foreskin that seems unusually tight or trapped.

These symptoms may indicate a medical condition where circumcision could be recommended.

VACCINES

Children are offered their booster vaccines at the age of four or five. These are usually administered in school but, in some areas, an appointment with the GP is needed.

For children in Ireland born before 1 October 2024, the vaccines offered are as follows:

- 4-in-1 vaccine: Protects against diphtheria, tetanus, pertussis (whooping cough), and polio.
- MMR vaccine: Protects against measles, mumps, and rubella.

Children born after 1 October 2024 will be offered the 4-in-1 when they start school, and the MMR vaccine will also contain the chickenpox vaccine, also known as the 'varicella' vaccine. This vaccine is called the MMRV vaccine.

Back when they were babies, they got these injections in their thighs, but now that they are older, they will get the vaccines in their upper arm. Of course, now that they are older, they may be a little apprehensive about getting an injection, so it is best to talk through what will happen and what they can expect. Don't say, 'It won't hurt at all', it's better to describe it as a 'little scratch'. The public-health team that comes to schools to give the vaccines are experts at their job and putting children at ease.

Your child may have a bit of pain and redness around the site of the injection, and it is fine to give them paracetamol or ibuprofen. Some children might also develop a fever, but this should resolve within 48 hours, and it is usually less than 38.5°C.

CONGRATULATIONS!

Your child is now five years old and will likely be starting 'big school'! All this talk of school is getting me emotional. Can you believe it? Your child went all the way from a toddler to going to school in three short years? The day you see them trotting off to school with their little backpack is so special. Cherish it.

All sorts of things happen in the first five years of your child's life. They reach milestones, build relationships, form memories, and lay the foundation of who they are going to be for the rest of their life.

Sometimes, there are bumps along the way, be those developmental differences or illnesses. The next section of this book is to help you if you do encounter these bumps in the road. It will help you to recognise any challenges or illnesses your child is facing and empower you to advocate for them.

PART II
Health Concerns in the Early Years

As parents, we try to do our best to ensure that our children are healthy and well. However, life has a funny way of being unpredictable, and this also applies to our babies' and children's health and development. Sometimes, our health concerns for our children are little niggles that just won't go away but, sometimes, they are immediate and urgent.

In this next section, I walk you through some common, and not so common, health concerns that you might have about your child's health. I will signpost who might be of help to you when you have concerns, and give you red flags for when you need to take urgent action.

The aim of this section is to equip you with the tools to recognise when something is amiss with your child's health or development, and to empower you to advocate for your child in healthcare settings.

CHAPTER 8
Tummy Troubles

When your toddler can express the pain they are feeling, there's a good chance that tummy pain will be top of the list. Tummy pain is one of the most common complaints in young children and one of the most frequent reasons parents seek medical advice. It can be brief and mild, or it can be persistent and worrying. It may accompany changes in pooping patterns, like diarrhoea or constipation, or there may be no other symptoms apart from your child saying, 'My tummy hurts.'

As a parent, it can be hard to know what's going on. Little children often can't describe exactly what they're feeling or where the pain is. They may cry, refuse food, or become clingier than usual. And because tummy pain can come from something as simple as needing to do a poo or as serious as a surgical emergency, it's understandable that it can cause you anxiety.

Let's take a look at the most common causes of tummy pain in toddlers and preschoolers, and how to recognise more serious symptoms.

COMMON CAUSES OF TUMMY PAIN

Constipation

The vast majority of tummy aches in young children are caused by temporary issues, and one of the most frequent culprits is constipation. Many parents are surprised to learn that a child can poo every day and still be constipated. In toddlers, constipation often means the child isn't fully emptying their bowels. This leads to a build-up of poo in the lower part of the colon, which stretches the bowel wall and causes pain. The discomfort may come and go, or it may seem to settle after the child finally manages to do a poo, only to return a few days later. Children who have recently started playschool or 'big' school may worry about using an unfamiliar toilet and withhold stool throughout the day. This can, in turn, lead to constipation.

To manage constipation, increase fibre-rich foods (fruit, vegetables, wholegrains) and encourage regular water intake to help keep stools soft. Giving your child relaxed, unhurried toilet time after meals can also encourage them to better empty their bowels. If the problem is ongoing, a GP may recommend a short course of stool-softening medication.

There is further discussion of causes and how you can help your child with constipation on page 204.

Trapped wind

Another common reason for tummy pain is trapped wind. Young children swallow air when they cry, eat quickly, or drink from bottles and sippy cups. If that air gets stuck in the digestive system, it can cause crampy, gassy discomfort.

Gentle tummy massage, bicycling your child's legs, or encouraging them to move around can help release trapped gas. Offering smaller, slower-paced meals and checking bottle teats for overly fast flow can reduce the amount of air swallowed.

Viral infections

Viral infections are another frequent cause of tummy discomfort. Viral gastroenteritis can lead to stomach cramps, vomiting, and diarrhoea. Often, the tummy pain begins before the vomiting starts, making it hard to realise that a virus is to blame. Even respiratory infections, such as colds and sore throats, can cause tummy pain, as the body's response to infection can involve lymph glands (also called nodes) in the tummy. Swollen lymph glands in the tummy are called 'mesenteric adenitis'. These glands can remain swollen for some time after an infection, meaning that the tummy pain can persist for several days or even weeks after a viral infection.

To manage viral infections, keep your child comfortable with rest and offer plenty of fluids to prevent dehydration, especially if vomiting or diarrhoea are present. Bland foods like toast, crackers, or banana when they're ready to eat are the most gentle options for the stomach. If symptoms worsen or your child becomes very lethargic, seek medical advice promptly.

Hunger or overeating

Young children may also get tummy pain from hunger or overeating. Many toddlers are grazers, snacking throughout the day, which can make it harder to notice hunger patterns. An empty stomach can feel uncomfortable, but so can a very full one, especially if the child eats too quickly.

Establishing a regular meal and snack routine can help prevent big swings between hunger and fullness. Encouraging your child to eat slowly and chew well can also reduce discomfort after meals.

Toddler diarrhoea

Toddler diarrhoea is a harmless but persistent condition where children have frequent loose stools, often several times a day, sometimes with undigested food in them. The poo is not usually watery like those in a tummy bug and the child is otherwise well and growing normally. Toddler diarrhoea does not typically cause severe tummy pain, but mild cramping or urgency to poo can be part of the picture.

Try reducing fruit juice and other high-sugar drinks, and offer more starchy foods like pasta, rice, and bread, to help firm up their poo. Keeping your child hydrated and ensuring a balanced diet will also support healthy digestion. See also page 206–207.

Functional abdominal pain

Lastly, and perhaps most difficult to understand, is functional abdominal pain. This is tummy pain that has no identifiable medical cause. It is very real to the child but is often linked to emotional or developmental factors. Even children as young as three can experience physical symptoms in response to stress or change. Starting preschool, adjusting to a new sibling, or navigating early toilet training can all contribute to these types of tummy aches.

The best approach is a calm and consistent response. Acknowledge that the pain is real, offer reassurance and listen to your child's concerns, as feeling understood can help reduce symptoms. Avoid giving rewards for not having pain or allowing the pain to prevent crèche or preschool attendance unless your child seems unwell.

Keeping a symptom diary can help spot patterns or triggers. Some families find it helpful to use simple relaxation techniques, tummy massage, or playful breathing games to support their child through these episodes. Keeping routines predictable and helping your child develop coping skills for change can make tummy pain episodes less frequent.

If the pain is severe, long-lasting, or interfering with daily life, your GP may refer you to a paediatrician or specialist for further support.

TUMMY PAIN AND EMOTIONS

Parents often ask whether anxiety can cause tummy pain in children, and the answer is yes. The connection between the gut and the brain is strong and well established. In adults, we often feel nervousness or fear in our stomachs, with sensations of butterflies or nausea. In children, emotional stress can show up as vague tummy discomfort.

By the age of three or four, many children begin to express their emotions through their bodies. A child who is worried about going to preschool may complain of a sore tummy every morning. The pain is not imagined; it is the child's way of expressing distress in the only language they know.

Understanding this connection helps avoid over-investigating symptoms and allows for gentle support. It's also why routines, sleep, and reassurance can play such an important role in helping children with ongoing tummy aches.

MORE SERIOUS CAUSES OF TUMMY PAIN

Although uncommon, there are a few conditions that can cause significant tummy pain in young children and need prompt medical attention.

- **Appendicitis:** This is one of the better-known causes of acute abdominal pain and can occur in children under five, although it is more typical from school age onwards. It often begins with pain around the belly button, followed by pain in the lower right part of the abdomen. Children may also have a fever, be off their food, vomit, or seem unusually tired.

- **Intussusception:** This is a rare condition where part of the intestine folds into itself like a telescope. This can cause waves of severe, cramping pain. The child may scream, pull up their legs, then go quiet, only for the pain to return again minutes later. Vomiting and red, jelly-like stools can also be a feature.
- **Testicular torsion:** While rare, this can present with lower tummy pain in boys, even as young as one. If your little boy is crying in pain and refusing to walk or stand, or you notice a swollen or red testicle, it is important to seek urgent medical advice. Torsion is a surgical emergency.
- **Coeliac disease:** This is another important cause of ongoing tummy trouble in young children. It is an autoimmune condition where the immune system reacts abnormally to gluten, a protein found in wheat, barley and rye. Rates of coeliac disease are particularly high in Ireland, likely due to a combination of genetic and environmental factors, so it's something doctors keep a close eye out for when tummy symptoms persist. In children with coeliac disease, eating gluten damages the lining of the small intestine, making it harder to absorb nutrients. Symptoms can include persistent diarrhoea or constipation, bloating, tummy pain, poor weight gain or weight loss, irritability, and fatigue. Some children may have no obvious tummy symptoms at all but show signs of nutritional deficiencies, such as anaemia or faltering growth. Coeliac disease can develop at any age after gluten is introduced to the diet, but it is often picked up between ages two and five. Diagnosis involves a blood test and, if positive, further assessment with a paediatrician. The only treatment is a strict, lifelong gluten-free diet, which usually leads to a full recovery and normal growth.

Other conditions that can cause abdominal pain include hernias and gallstones, though these are all relatively uncommon in children. Pain from a urinary tract infection may not be obvious in its location and instead present with fever, irritability, or a refusal to eat. New onset type 1 diabetes can present with tummy pain.

Most tummy pain in children settles within a few hours or a couple of days and improves with simple measures.

However, the following are signs that suggest the need for medical advice:

- persistent or worsening pain over several days
- pain that wakes a child at night
- vomiting that doesn't settle or includes bile (green fluid)
- blood in the poo or vomit
- a distended or very tender tummy
- high fever (over 38°C) with pain
- lethargy or unusual drowsiness
- pain that is always in the same place
- weight loss or failure to gain weight
- reduced urine production (dehydration)
- increased urine production (can mean type 1 diabetes)
- behavioural changes such as withdrawal or unusual irritability.

Trust your instincts. If something doesn't feel right, speak to your GP or attend an out-of-hours GP service or emergency department, depending on the severity.

UNDERSTANDING CONSTIPATION

Constipation is the most common underlying cause of chronic tummy pain in young children. It is often missed because the child may still be passing some stools, but not enough to fully empty their bowels. This partial evacuation can lead to a stretched bowel, which becomes sluggish and less sensitive over time.

Signs of constipation include hard or painful stools, large poos that block the toilet, stool withholding behaviours such as crossing the legs or tiptoeing, a bloated tummy, and soiling or small leaks of poo in the pants. Soiling is not a behavioural problem; it is usually a sign that there is a build-up of poo, and softer poo is leaking around it without the child having much control.

If a child has just two of the following symptoms, they may be constipated.

- passing stool types 1–3 on the Bristol Stool Chart (see page 205)
- passing fewer than four poos per week
- passing three or more poos per day (this can mean a full bowel, with poo leaking out)
- soiling (this can be soft or hard, and the child has no control over it)
- passing occasional very large poos
- pain on pooing
- a distended tummy
- smelly poo or wind or bad breath
- nausea
- urine problems related to frequency, wetting, or urine infections.

A really good way to help detect constipation in your child is to use the Bristol Stool Chart.

Type	Description	Meaning	
1	Separate hard lumps, like nuts	Constipation	
2	Sausage-shaped but lumpy	Mild constipation	
3	Like a sausage with cracks	Slightly dry but generally normal	
4	Smooth, soft sausage or snake	Ideal / healthy stool	
5	Soft blobs with clear edges	Loose stool / mild diarrhoea	
6	Fluffy pieces with ragged edges, mushy	Diarrhoea	
7	Watery, no solid pieces	Severe diarrhoea	

How to help

Helping a child with constipation starts with a good toilet routine. Timing is important: if your child is constipated, sit them on the loo or potty 20–30 minutes after a meal for 10–15 minutes. It is usually easier to poop if the child is sitting in a position where the knees rest slightly above the hips. This is easy on a potty, but it needs some thought when it comes to the 'big' toilet. A child-sized toilet seat and footstool can help them sit comfortably and enable the bowel to empty more effectively.

Ensure your child has plenty of water throughout the day and offer high-fibre foods, such as fruit, vegetables, and wholegrains. Avoid overloading with fruit juices, which can sometimes make things worse. Sometimes, dietary changes alone aren't enough and a gentle laxative, such as macrogol (often prescribed as Movicol in Ireland and the UK), may be recommended. This is safe and effective for children but it should always be used with medical guidance, especially if constipation has been long-standing.

An excellent resource for all things pee- and poo-related is ERIC: The Children's Bowel & Bladder Charity (www.eric.org.uk).

Toilet training and constipation

The age at which toilet training begins varies widely, but many children start showing interest between two and three years old. While toilet training does not directly cause constipation, pressure around using the toilet can contribute to stool withholding and anxiety. If a child has one painful poo, they may decide not to go next time. This leads to more drying and hardening of the stool, more discomfort, and a cycle that can be difficult to break.

A relaxed, child-led approach to toilet training is best. Encourage, don't push. Praise sitting on the potty or toilet, even if no poo comes. Avoid punishment or expressions of frustration. If your child develops constipation during toilet training, it's often wise to take a step back and try again a few weeks later.

UNDERSTANDING TODDLER DIARRHOEA

Toddler diarrhoea is a common and completely benign condition in children aged between one and five years. It is not caused by infection or allergy, and it is not a sign of a serious problem.

The main feature is frequent loose stools, often with bits of undigested food, but the child is otherwise growing well and feeling fine.

The likely explanation is that food moves through the bowel too quickly. This gives the gut less time to absorb water, resulting in looser stools. Contributing factors may include a diet that is low in fat and high in fibre or sugar, as well as excess fruit juice or squash.

The treatment for toddler diarrhoea is simple: reduce fruit juice and sweet drinks, limit excessive fruit, and ensure your child is eating regular meals that include some fat. Foods such as full-fat yogurt, cheese, peanut butter, and avocado are helpful. Avoid giving anti-diarrhoeal medication as this is not suitable for young children.

One of my toddlers had toddler diarrhoea and I discovered that the culprit was raisins! It made sense – raisins are high in sugar and fibre. It is different for every toddler though, so speak to your GP before you start eliminating foods from your child's diet.

Most children grow out of toddler diarrhoea by school age, and no treatment is usually needed beyond dietary adjustments and reassurance.

WHAT IF THERE IS NO OBVIOUS CAUSE OF TUMMY PAIN?

Sometimes, after all the tests are done and the diet has been reviewed, your child still complains of tummy pain. This may be what doctors call 'functional abdominal pain', which is pain that has no identifiable cause and may be linked to emotional or developmental factors (see page 200).

HELPING YOUR CHILD TALK ABOUT TUMMY PAIN

Toddlers and preschoolers may not have the language to explain what they feel, so you can help by observing behaviour and using simple words. Ask whether it feels 'squeezy', 'pinching', 'hurty', or 'like needing a poo'. Some children respond well to visuals, such as pointing to pictures of body parts or using books about digestion.

Keep the tone relaxed. Avoid overfocusing on the pain or asking too many questions. Sometimes, attention can unintentionally reinforce the symptom – instead, offer reassurance, distraction, and connection.

Tummy pain in young children is common and usually not serious. Whether it's a case of trapped wind, constipation, toddler diarrhoea, or functional tummy pain, most children recover quickly with time, reassurance, and some simple changes to diet and routine.

However, there are times when tummy pain can be a sign of something more serious. Knowing what signs to watch out for and when to seek medical advice can help you feel confident in managing your little one's tummy troubles.

CHAPTER 9
Developmental Differences

As you will have learned already from this book, babies, toddlers, and children develop at their own unique pace. However, you might notice patterns in your child that make you wonder whether they are facing developmental challenges in particular areas. You may have done some research online and come across terms such as 'neurodivergent', 'autism', 'dyspraxia', or 'ADHD' and wondered if these might apply to your child.

If you are in this situation, it is very natural to feel anxious and overwhelmed. Please remember that your GP and your public-health nurse are a good place to start when looking for guidance about possible developmental challenges or delays.

WHAT IS NEURODIVERGENCE?

'Neurodivergence' is a non-medical term used to describe variations in the human brain regarding learning, attention, mood, and other cognitive functions. These variations are not 'disorders'; rather, they are different ways of experiencing and interacting with the world.

Coined in the 1990s by sociologist Judy Singer, the term 'neurodiversity' aims to reduce stigma and promote acceptance of individuals who think and perceive differently. When a child is neurodivergent, it means their brain works differently from what is considered 'neurotypical'.

Neurodivergence includes a range of conditions, such as:

- sensory processing disorder (SPD)
- dyspraxia (developmental co-ordination disorder)
- attention deficit (hyperactivity) disorder (ADD/ADHD)
- autism spectrum disorder (ASD)
- learning difficulties, such as dyslexia and dyscalculia.

This chapter will focus on those conditions that commonly appear in children aged one to five.

SENSORY PROCESSING DISORDER (SPD)

AMELIA'S STORY

Amelia, aged three, would scream and run away whenever her mother tried to brush her hair. She refused to wear certain clothes, especially those with tags or tight necklines, and she covered her ears at the sound of the vacuum cleaner. Her nursery teacher noticed that she struggled to sit still at story time and preferred solitary play. With guidance from an occupational therapist, Amelia's parents learned to use a 'sensory diet' (a structured activity plan) that helped regulate her sensory needs.

Sensory processing disorder refers to the brain's difficulty receiving and responding to information from the senses.

Children with SPD may be overly sensitive to stimuli (hypersensitive), under-responsive (hyposensitive), or show a mix of both.

Signs of SPD in toddlers and preschoolers include:

- an overreaction to textures, noises, lights, or smells
- difficulty with grooming activities (e.g. brushing teeth or washing hair)
- constant movement or, conversely, seeming unusually still
- the avoidance of certain textures or types of play (e.g. messy play).

DYSPRAXIA (DEVELOPMENTAL CO-ORDINATION DISORDER)

> ### LIAM'S STORY
> Liam, aged four, had trouble using cutlery and couldn't pedal his tricycle, even though many of his peers could. He often spilled drinks and fell more frequently than other children. His parents were concerned and, after assessment by a paediatrician and an occupational therapist, Liam was diagnosed with dyspraxia. A targeted therapy plan helped improve his motor planning and co-ordination, and he began to grow more confident in physical activities.

Dyspraxia affects motor-skill development and co-ordination. It can also impact speech, memory, and organisation.

Signs of dyspraxia in young children include:

- a delay in reaching motor milestones (e.g. crawling or walking)
- difficulty with activities that require co-ordination (e.g. catching a ball or using utensils)
- trouble with speech clarity
- challenges with toilet training
- frequent tripping or bumping into things.

ADD/ADHD

> ### JACK'S STORY
>
> Jack, a lively four-year-old, was always on the move. He struggled to sit during mealtimes and had difficulty following instructions in his preschool. He often interrupted others and had a hard time waiting his turn. After consultation with his GP and referral to a child psychologist, Jack was diagnosed with ADHD. With behavioural strategies at home and support from his preschool staff, Jack began to thrive in structured environments.

Attention deficit disorder (ADD) and attention deficit hyperactivity disorder (ADHD) are characterised by difficulties with attention, impulsivity, and, in some cases, hyperactivity. ADHD is commonly diagnosed in school-aged children, but it can show signs as early as toddlerhood.

Signs of ADD/ADHD in preschoolers include:

- constant motion and difficulty sitting still
- trouble focusing on tasks or play

- impulsive behaviour (e.g. grabbing toys, difficulty waiting)
- frequent emotional outbursts
- seeming 'not to listen', even when spoken to directly
- risk-taking behaviour or seeming unaware of danger.

AUTISM

> ### SOPHIE'S STORY
> Sophie, aged three, rarely responded to her name and preferred lining up her toys over interactive play. She used few words and became distressed when her routine changed. After seeing a speech therapist and undergoing a developmental assessment through her local services, Sophie was diagnosed with autism. Her family accessed support from an early-intervention programme and began using visual supports to aid communication.

Autism is a neurodevelopmental condition that affects communication, social interaction, and behaviour. Autism exists on a spectrum, meaning every child is different. Some children may have what is referred to as 'Level 1' autism (requiring minimal support), while others may have more complex needs (Level 2 or 3), including co-occurring intellectual disabilities.

Children with autism and an intellectual disability may have significantly delayed language, and daily-living and cognitive skills. They may require more extensive support across settings. Conversely, some autistic children have average or above-average intellectual abilities, and they struggle mainly with social communication or sensory processing.

Signs of autism in children aged one to five include:

- limited eye contact or reduced facial expressions
- delayed speech or language regression
- preference for routines and distress at changes
- intense interest in particular topics or objects
- repetitive behaviours (e.g. hand-flapping, rocking)
- limited interest in peers or pretend play.

Myths about autism

Despite growing awareness, many myths and misconceptions about autism persist. Listed here are a few common ones.

Myth 1 – 'All autistic children are non-speaking':
- In reality, autism is a spectrum. Some children may have limited speech, while others may speak fluently but have difficulty with social communication.

Myth 2 – 'Autism is caused by bad parenting or emotional trauma':
- There is no evidence to support this. Autism is a neurodevelopmental condition likely caused by a mix of genetic and environmental factors.

Myth 3 – 'Children with autism don't make friends':
- Many autistic children desire friendship, but they may struggle with the social skills needed to connect. With support, they can build meaningful relationships.

Myth 4 – 'You can grow out of autism':
- Autism is lifelong. Children don't outgrow it, but, with the right support, they can develop skills that will help them thrive.

Myth 5 – 'All autistic people have savant skills':
- While some may have remarkable abilities in specific areas, this is not typical of all autistic individuals.

Myth 6 – 'Vaccines cause autism':
- This is one of the most widespread and damaging myths. Extensive research across many countries, including Ireland and the UK, has shown no link between vaccines (including the MMR vaccine) and autism. The original study that sparked concern was retracted because of serious ethical violations and flawed data. Major health organisations – including the HSE, NHS, World Health Organization, and the Royal College of Paediatrics and Child Health – strongly support the safety and importance of childhood vaccinations. Vaccines protect children from serious and potentially life-threatening illnesses.

WHAT ARE EARLY SIGNS OF NEURODIVERGENCE?

Parents are usually the first to notice when something seems different. Trust your instincts. Some early signs that may warrant a closer look include:

- a lack of babbling or gesturing by 12 months
- no single words by 16 months
- no two-word phrases by 24 months
- loss of language or social skills at any age
- infrequent eye contact
- limited interest in other children
- heightened sensitivity or indifference to pain, textures, or noise
- difficulty with transitions or new routines
- delayed motor skills.

Getting a diagnosis

You do not need a diagnosis to begin accessing support. Early intervention is the key and there are some steps you can take if you have concerns.

Step 1: Observe and document your concerns
You may notice that your child is:

- not meeting milestones (such as crawling, talking, or making eye contact)
- struggling with communication or interaction
- repeating behaviours (e.g. hand flapping, lining up toys)
- seeming unusually sensitive to sounds or touch.

These can be early signs of developmental differences, so start by noting specific behaviours, how often they occur, and anything that seems to trigger or calm your child.

Step 2: Speak to your GP
Your first formal step is to book an appointment with your GP, who can:

- listen to your concerns
- carry out initial screenings
- refer your child for further assessment, if needed.

If your child is under five, your GP may refer you to the children's disability network team. For older children or those with fewer support needs, you may be referred to primary-care services or other appropriate specialists.

Step 3: Involve your public-health nurse
If your child is under school age, your local public-health nurse can be a helpful ally. They may pick up developmental concerns

during routine check-ups or can help you access services through the HSE.

Step 4: Request an Assessment of Need (if under five)
Under the Irish Disability Act 2005, you can apply for an Assessment of Need through your local HSE office. This formal process:

- evaluates whether your child has a disability
- identifies what services are required (e.g. speech therapy or occupational therapy).

You must apply for this assessment before your child turns five.

Step 5: Assessments and therapy
Depending on the outcome of referrals, your child may undergo further evaluations by:

- speech-and-language therapists
- occupational therapists
- psychologists
- developmental paediatricians.

Early Intervention Services (for 0–5 years) and School-Age Disability Services (for 5+) can also provide co-ordinated support.

Step 6: Engage with the school system
If your child is in preschool or primary school:

- speak with the teacher or principal about your concerns
- request that the school involve a special education needs organiser (SENO) to arrange additional supports (such as a special needs assistant (SNA) or a special class).

The National Educational Psychological Service (NEPS) can also provide psychological assessments and guidance.

Step 7: Connect with parent support networks

Parenting a child with additional needs can feel isolating, but you are not alone. Many national and local organisations offer practical advice and emotional support. These include:

- AsIAm, Ireland's national autism charity
- Inclusion Ireland, which advocates for people with intellectual disabilities
- Irish Society for Autism
- Rare Ireland, a charity for children with rare genetic conditions.

These groups often offer workshops, peer support, and help navigating services.

IS THERE SOMETHING MORE GOING ON?

The majority of children with developmental differences have no underlying health problems. However, sometimes developmental delays can be a sign of an underlying neurological or genetic condition.

Your child may have physical traits of a possible underlying diagnosis, or your GP, public-health nurse, or community team may have queries. In this case, you may be referred to a paediatrician or paediatric neurologist, who may recommend specialised tests, such as genetic blood tests or certain types of brain scans.

SUPPORTING YOUR CHILD AT HOME

There can be a lot of tests involved when your child receives a diagnosis, paperwork to take care of, and, frustratingly, long waiting lists for appointments. While you are navigating the route to diagnosis and support, there are some things you can be doing at home to help your child to thrive:

- Establish predictable routines: Children feel more secure when they know what to expect.
- Use visual supports: Picture schedules (a visual schedule for upcoming events) can ease transitions.
- Break down tasks: Simplify steps and celebrate small achievements.
- Encourage play: All children learn through play – follow your child's interests.
- Practise gentle communication: Use clear, calm language.
- Minimise overwhelm: Create quiet spaces and avoid sensory overload.
- Focus on strengths: Celebrate what your child can do and loves to do.

WHAT IF NO ONE HEARS MY CONCERNS?

As a parent, you are your child's most consistent and important advocate. Navigating developmental differences can be overwhelming but, remember, you are not alone and your instincts matter. You know your child best.

Some parents worry about seeming overanxious or being dismissed but, if something feels different, it's okay to keep asking questions. Sometimes, it takes multiple visits or conversations before concerns are fully understood or acted on. That's not a reflection of your parenting; it's a reflection of how complex child development can be.

Your persistence in seeking answers is a strength, not a flaw. If you feel unheard, consider seeking a second opinion.

The early years matter. Early support, whether or not you have a formal diagnosis, can make a big difference. You don't have to wait for a diagnosis to start making helpful changes at home or to seek guidance.

Remember, neurodivergence is not a deficit; it is a difference. With the right support, all children can thrive.

CHAPTER 10
Is This Something Serious?

As parents, many of us have experienced brief moments of fear that something serious might be going on with our child's health. Thankfully, most of the time our concerns are put to rest, either by symptoms resolving or healthcare professionals going through our concerns with us and providing reassurance.

But, sometimes, those niggles and concerns do not go away, and the signs mount up that there may be something serious going on. So, how do you best advocate for your child when you are really worried that an urgent health situation is emerging?

Most childhood illnesses are harmless and clear up quickly. But, sometimes, a more serious condition starts off looking very similar to everyday bugs or tiredness. This chapter will help you recognise the signs that something might need a closer look, and we will cover serious long-term health conditions, such as type 1 diabetes, epilepsy, and childhood cancer.

Please note that if you are concerned about your child suddenly deteriorating in the context of a viral or bacterial illness, this may be sepsis, which is an acute medical emergency that you can read more about on page 357.

WHAT'S NORMAL AND WHAT'S NOT

What we usually see in everyday illness includes:

- coughs, colds, or mild fevers that settle in a few days
- temporary tiredness or fussiness
- a couple of days off food because of a bug
- brief tummy upsets, earaches, or sore throats.

Some signs that deserve a second look include:

- symptoms that last more than a week without improving
- a child who is increasingly tired or pale
- unusual or frequent bruising
- lumps or swollen glands that don't go away
- unexplained fevers or night sweats
- unexplained weight loss
- new problems with balance, behaviour, or vision.

If you feel uneasy about how your child is, even if it's hard to explain, that alone is reason to check in with your GP.

TYPE 1 DIABETES

ANNA'S STORY

Nina noticed her daughter, Anna, was needing the toilet a lot more than usual and asking for drinks constantly. She started wetting the bed, having previously been dry at night. She'd also become thinner over the previous few weeks. She was exhausted, and although she was four, she had gone back to taking a nap in the afternoon. The GP checked Anna's urine and found that it contained glucose. Normally, glucose is not present in the urine,

> but when blood glucose levels are high, it leaks into the urine. Anna's blood glucose level was very high. Anna was sent straight to the emergency department, where she was diagnosed with type 1 diabetes and admitted to hospital to start treatment.

Type 1 diabetes is an autoimmune condition in which the immune system mistakenly attacks and destroys the insulin-producing beta cells in the pancreas. Without insulin, the body cannot regulate blood glucose levels, which can lead to serious health complications if left untreated. It is distinct from type 2 diabetes, which is more often linked to lifestyle factors and typically occurs in adults.

Type 1 diabetes often develops rapidly over a few days or weeks. Classic symptoms include:

- increased thirst (polydipsia) and urination (polyuria)
- extreme tiredness or fatigue
- weight loss, despite normal or increased appetite
- fruity-smelling breath (a sign of ketones, a byproduct of the way the body's metabolism compensates for not being able to absorb sugar properly)
- blurred vision
- mood changes or irritability
- thrush or slow-healing infections
- bedwetting in a previously dry child, or waking frequently at night to pee.

If diabetes is not identified early symptoms can escalate to diabetic ketoacidosis, a medical emergency characterised by vomiting, abdominal pain, rapid breathing, and confusion.

If you suspect your child may have type 1 diabetes, seek urgent medical attention. Early diagnosis can prevent serious complications.

> **REMEMBER THE FIVE Ts:**
> - Toilet: going more often, especially at night
> - Thirsty: drinking a lot
> - Tired: noticeably more fatigued
> - Thinner: losing weight without trying
> - Tummy: pain or discomfort, vomiting.

What causes type 1 diabetes?

The exact cause is not fully understood, but type 1 diabetes is believed to be triggered by a combination of genetic and environmental factors:

- Genetics: A family history of type 1 diabetes slightly increases risk, although most children who are diagnosed have no close relatives with the condition. However, there may be a family history of other autoimmune conditions (e.g. coeliac disease, hypothyroidism).
- Autoimmunity: The immune system mistakenly targets insulin-producing cells.
- Environmental triggers: Viruses and other unknown factors may initiate the autoimmune process.

It is important to note that type 1 diabetes is not caused by lifestyle or diet and cannot be prevented.

Diagnosis

Diagnosis is usually made by a GP or hospital paediatrician, often following an emergency presentation. Diagnosis typically involves:

- blood glucose tests to confirm elevated blood sugar levels
- urine tests to check for ketones and glucose
- a HbA1c test to assess average blood sugar over recent months
- autoantibody tests to confirm the autoimmune nature of the condition.

Treatment of type 1 diabetes is to replace the insulin the pancreas can no longer produce. Insulin is administered via injection, and blood sugar levels are monitored closely. The introduction of insulin pumps and continuous glucose monitors has had a very positive impact on the treatment of diabetes.

Living with type 1 diabetes

Children with type 1 diabetes can lead full, active lives. With good control, they can participate in school, sports, and social activities like any other child. Key aspects of long-term care include:

- regular diabetes reviews (eye exams, kidney tests, foot checks)
- support during puberty and transition to adult care
- mental-health support to manage the emotional impact of the diagnosis.

Prognosis and outlook

While type 1 diabetes is a serious condition, modern treatments mean that children with it can thrive. With effective management:

- short-term risks, like hypoglycaemia and diabetic ketoacidosis, can be minimised
- long-term complications (kidney disease, eye problems, cardiovascular issues) are greatly reduced through good glucose control.

Medical advancements and research into immune therapies continue to improve the quality of life and outcomes for those living with type 1 diabetes.

EPILEPSY

> ### ISLA'S STORY: CHILDHOOD ABSENCE EPILEPSY
>
> At first, Matt thought his seven-year-old daughter, Isla, was just daydreaming. She'd stare off for a few seconds, sometimes flutter her eyelids, and then carry on like nothing happened. Her teachers noticed that she didn't seem to be paying attention as well as usual in school and said they were worried about her. So, Isla's parents brought her to the GP, who referred them to a paediatrician for review. While they were waiting for their appointment, they managed to video some of the episodes that were concerning them. This was very helpful for the paediatrician, who then arranged further tests.

> ### PADDY'S STORY: FOCAL SEIZURES WITH AWARENESS
>
> Seven-year-old Paddy started to have short episodes every few days where his mouth felt strange, and the right-hand side of his face would twitch for about 20 seconds. No matter how hard he tried, he could not stop the twitches.

> During one of these episodes, he went to find his mum. 'It was so strange,' recalls Mary. 'He was looking at me, fully alert, but he couldn't talk, and he couldn't stop the twitching.' Mary got her phone out and recorded the last few seconds, then brought Paddy straight to the GP. They were then sent to the hospital. The video recording Mary took of Paddy's seizure was really useful to the doctors and nurses, as it helped them to make the diagnosis.

> ### KATIE'S STORY: TONIC-CLONIC SEIZURES
>
> Nine-year-old Katie suddenly stiffened and fell to the floor. Then, her arms and legs started jerking, and her eyes rolled. She couldn't hear her parents or respond to them. 'It was terrifying,' said Rachel. 'We didn't know if it was a seizure, a faint, or something else.' Rachel called 999 and the paramedics attended to Katie. She was brought by ambulance to the emergency department where she was assessed and then discharged home, with advice to Rachel to follow up with Katie's GP. The emergency doctors also made a referral for follow-up with a paediatric neurologist.

Epilepsy is a condition where a child has repeated seizures due to sudden bursts of electrical activity in the brain. It's more common than many people realise, with around 1 in every 200 children in Ireland and the UK having epilepsy.

As you can see from Isla's, Paddy's, and Katie's stories, seizures can look very different from child to child. Not all involve collapsing or shaking; some are subtle and easy to miss at first. Epilepsy can involve focal (partial) seizures, which start in one part of the brain, or generalised seizures, which affect both sides of the brain at once.

The following are the common types of seizures seen in children.

Absence seizures (petit mal)
- Sudden staring spells lasting 5–15 seconds.
- May involve blinking or slight facial twitching.
- Often mistaken for daydreaming or inattention.
- Child is unaware during the event.

Focal seizures with awareness
- Strange sensations (smells, tastes, déjà vu).
- Twitching in one part of the body.
- Child may be able to speak or respond.

Focal seizures with impaired awareness
- Staring, unresponsiveness, and chewing or picking motions.
- Lasts 30 seconds to a few minutes.
- Often followed by confusion or tiredness.

Tonic-clonic seizures (what most people imagine)
- Stiffening of limbs, followed by jerking.
- Loss of consciousness.
- May involve drooling, bladder/bowel release.
- Often followed by sleepiness or confusion (post-ictal phase).

Infantile spasms

I will mention infantile spasms (IS) here as well, even though they are not common. These are a *rare* type of epilepsy that affect babies under the age of one, but they are serious, and early recognition is very important. During an infantile spasm, babies:

- suddenly stiffen or startle
- flex their body forward
- arch their back.

These movements occur in clusters of up to 50 spasms, usually as the baby is waking or falling asleep.

At around the same time as babies with IS start to have spasms, they often show signs of developmental regression. They may stop rolling over or sitting, they may become withdrawn and stop smiling or babbling, or they may become very irritable. It is very important to treat IS early, as they can have a significant impact on a baby's development. If you suspect your baby has infantile spasms, seek medical attention urgently.

What to do if your child has a seizure

Seeing your child have a seizure can be frightening. Whether it's a generalised seizure (whole-body shaking, loss of consciousness) or a focal seizure (twitching or unusual movements in just one area, staring, or unresponsiveness), staying calm and knowing what to do can make a big difference.

Step 1: Keep your child safe
- Lay them gently on the ground or on a safe surface.
- Move any hard or sharp objects to prevent injury.
- Place something soft under their head if possible.
- If they are on the ground, roll them onto their side after the shaking stops (or immediately if they are vomiting or have lots of saliva) to help keep their airway clear.
- Do not put anything in their mouth – it will not stop tongue-biting and may cause harm.
- Loosen tight clothing around the neck.

Step 2: Observe and record
If you can, take note of the following:

- how long the seizure lasts (use your phone's timer)
- any colour changes, especially blueness around the lips
- if your child wet themselves during the episode
- what happened before the seizure (were they ill, tired, upset, or did they have an unusual sensation?)
- how they behaved afterwards (confused, sleepy, or back to normal quickly).

If possible, video the seizure on your phone – this can be extremely helpful for doctors in making a diagnosis.

Step 3: Know when to call 999
Call emergency services straightaway if any of the following occurs:

- the seizure lasts more than five minutes
- it's their first seizure
- they have repeated seizures without regaining consciousness in between
- they have difficulty breathing after the seizure
- they are injured during the seizure
- the seizure happens in water
- they remain unconscious or unresponsive for a prolonged time afterwards
- they have another serious medical condition (e.g. heart problems, diabetes) and you are concerned.

Step 4: Know when to see a doctor
You should still contact your GP or specialist promptly for follow-up if your child:

- has had seizures before and this episode is typical for them
- recovers fully within minutes and is breathing normally
- is alert, responsive, and acting as they normally would after a short rest.

What to do after the first seizure

If your child has had what might be a seizure, whether it's a dramatic collapse or a short, strange episode, here are the next steps to take:

- See your GP if the episode was brief and your child has recovered. The GP may request blood tests or refer you to a paediatrician or neurologist.
- If needed, go to the emergency department, especially if your child is unconscious, the seizure lasts more than five minutes, they have breathing problems, or you're unsure.
- Keep a record. Note down what you saw, how long it lasted, and what happened before and after. It helps more than you might think.
- Start a seizure diary. Use your phone or a notebook to track events.

Preparing for a neurology appointment

Your neurology appointment will involve detailed questions about what's been happening. Your child doesn't need to have symptoms at the appointment, but videos and records help fill the gaps.

Coming prepared can be really helpful, so, if possible, make note of and bring the following:

- Videos: If you can, record any unusual episodes – even a short clip is very helpful.
- Diary entries: Include the date, time, what happened, how

long the episode lasted, and what your child was doing before and after the seizure.
- Possible triggers: Was your child tired, unwell, seeing flashing lights, stressed? Had they missed meals?
- Medical history: Note any past head injuries, infections, or family history of epilepsy.
- Questions: Write them down; it's easy to forget in the moment.

After your appointment, further tests, such as a brain scan and a recording of brain activity (an EEG), may be recommended. Depending on the results, treatment with antiseizure medication may be advised.

Prognosis and outlook

There is a good outlook for most children with epilepsy. Many outgrow it or achieve good control with medication. With proper management, most children can live active, fulfilling lives, including attending school, sports, and social activities. Regular follow-ups with a paediatric neurologist and/or epilepsy team are key.

Causes of epilepsy vary greatly, but it is important to remember that there is nothing a parent can do to prevent their child from developing epilepsy.

LEUKAEMIA

MARK'S STORY

Mark had been pale for a while and his mum, Tanya, noticed that he seemed to get every bug going. When he started complaining that his legs hurt and got a few bruises on his face that didn't make sense, she brought him to the GP. A blood test led to a referral to hospital.

Leukaemia is the most common type of childhood cancer, accounting for around a third of all cancers in children under 15. As a parent, the idea of your child facing such a diagnosis is deeply unsettling, but the treatment for leukaemia has advanced hugely in recent years and the prognosis for most children is very good.

Leukaemia is a cancer of the blood-forming tissues, including the bone marrow and lymphatic system. It causes the body to produce large numbers of abnormal white blood cells that don't function properly, crowding out healthy cells, and making it harder for the body to fight infections, stop bleeding, or carry oxygen.

There are two main types of leukaemia in children:

- Acute lymphoblastic leukaemia (ALL): the most common type in children.
- Acute myeloid leukaemia (AML): less common but still significant.

If your child has leukaemia, they might show the following signs:

- ongoing tiredness or sleepiness
- looking unusually pale
- bruising more easily or small red spots on the skin
- repeated infections or slow recovery
- aches in bones or joints
- enlarged glands or tummy.

What causes leukaemia?

The exact cause of most childhood leukaemia is still not fully understood. Unlike many adult cancers, lifestyle and environmental factors seem to play a much smaller role. There are some potential contributing factors:

- Genetic predisposition: certain genetic conditions (such as Down syndrome) are linked with a higher risk.

- Radiation or chemical exposure: although this is very rare in Ireland and the UK.
- Immune-system disorders: these may alter the body's cell production.

There is nothing a parent can do to prevent childhood leukaemia.

How is leukaemia diagnosed?

If a GP suspects your child has leukaemia, they will refer them to hospital for urgent tests, which may include:

- blood tests to check for abnormal levels of white cells, red cells, and platelets
- a bone-marrow biopsy, the definitive test where a small sample of bone marrow is taken, usually from the hip, to examine under a microscope
- a lumbar puncture to check if the cancer has spread to the fluid around the brain and spinal cord
- imaging, such as X-rays or ultrasounds, to look for swollen organs or lymph nodes.

In Ireland and the UK, children with suspected leukaemia are fast-tracked for diagnosis and treatment through paediatric oncology networks, such as the NHS Children's Cancer and Leukaemia Group (CCLG) and Children's Health Ireland (CHI).

Prognosis and outlook

Thanks to major advancements in treatment over recent decades, the prognosis for childhood leukaemia has greatly improved:

- ALL: Over 90% of children now survive five years or more after diagnosis.

- AML: The survival rate continues to improve, with around 70–80% long-term survival in children.

Factors that influence prognosis include the child's age, white-blood-cell count at diagnosis, genetic markers of the leukaemia cells, and how well the cancer responds to treatment.

LYMPHOMA

> ### JAMES'S STORY
> Ellie first noticed a lump on her son James's neck when she was drying his hair. He'd had a cold the week before, so she assumed it was just a swollen gland. But it didn't go away. Over the next three weeks it became larger and could be seen clearly on his neck. Ellie brought James to the GP, who examined the lump and decided to refer James to the local hospital for urgent review with the paediatric team. James had a lot of tests done and was diagnosed with lymphoma.

Lymphoma is a type of cancer that affects the lymphatic system, a crucial part of the immune system. While it is one of the more common childhood cancers, it's still relatively rare. The outcome after treatment is usually excellent.

Lymphoma is a cancer of the lymphocytes, a type of white blood cell that helps the body fight infections. It typically begins in the lymph nodes but can spread to other parts of the lymphatic system, including the spleen, bone marrow, thymus, and even the brain or spinal cord.

There are two main types of childhood lymphoma:

- Hodgkin lymphoma (HL).
- Non-Hodgkin lymphoma (NHL).

Both types have different characteristics and treatment protocols, but they share similar early symptoms.

Symptoms can develop gradually or suddenly. Many signs are non-specific and may mimic common infections, making early detection challenging. Things to look out for include:

- swollen lymph nodes, especially in the neck, armpits, or groin – these may be painless and persist without signs of infection
- persistent fever without an obvious cause
- night sweats
- unexplained weight loss
- fatigue and lethargy
- coughing or breathing difficulties (if lymph nodes in the chest are affected)
- abdominal pain or swelling
- itchy skin or rash
- frequent infections.

Swollen lymph nodes are very common in children, usually triggered by infections, such as colds or sore throats. However, there are important differences between reactive nodes (from infection) and lymphoma nodes.

Feature	Reactive Nodes (Infection)	Lymphoma Nodes
Tenderness	Often tender or painful	Usually painless
Size	Smaller, often less than 2 cm	Often larger than 2 cm
Mobility	Move freely under the skin	May feel fixed or firm

Feature	Reactive Nodes (Infection)	Lymphoma Nodes
Duration	Improve within 2–3 weeks	Persist or grow over time
Associated illness	Cold, sore throat, etc. present	May occur without infection

You should take your child to your GP if:

- a lymph node remains swollen for more than two or three weeks
- the swelling gets larger or feels hard or rubbery
- there are accompanying fevers, night sweats, weight loss, or fatigue
- you have any concerns about unexplained symptoms.

What causes childhood lymphoma?

The exact cause is unknown, but several factors may increase the risk:

- viral infections, such as Epstein-Barr virus (EBV)
- genetic conditions, such as ataxia-telangiectasia or Down syndrome.

There is nothing a parent can do to prevent childhood lymphoma.

How is lymphoma diagnosed?

Lymphoma is diagnosed in hospital, and early referral to a paediatric oncology team ensures prompt and accurate diagnosis. Several tests need to be done to confirm lymphoma, including:

- a physical examination to assess lymph nodes and general health

- blood tests to check white-cell counts and organ function
- imaging, such as X-ray, ultrasound, CT, or MRI scans, to locate enlarged nodes or masses
- a biopsy to take a small sample of lymph node tissue and examine it under a microscope
- a bone-marrow test to check if cancer has spread
- a PET scan, which is often used in Hodgkin lymphoma to assess spread and treatment response.

Prognosis and outlook

Thanks to advances in treatment, most children with lymphoma are cured:

- Hodgkin lymphoma: Over 90% survival rate.
- Non-Hodgkin lymphoma: Around 80–90% survival, depending on type and stage.

Prognosis improves with early diagnosis and access to specialist care. Most children go on to live long and healthy lives.

BRAIN TUMOURS

ELLA'S STORY

Ella, aged five, had been complaining of headaches, usually in the morning. Her mum, Anne, noticed she sometimes seemed off-balance and more irritable than usual. Then, she started vomiting and complaining of double vision. Anne was very worried about her daughter and brought her to the local emergency department where she underwent a brain scan, which diagnosed a tumour.

Brain tumours are the most common solid tumours (tumours that grow in a body organ as opposed to the blood or lymph nodes) in children and the second most common type of childhood cancer after leukaemia. While the diagnosis is rare and frightening, awareness of symptoms and advances in treatment can make a significant difference.

A brain tumour is an abnormal growth of cells in the brain or central nervous system. These can be:

- benign (non-cancerous), which are slower growing and less likely to spread
- malignant (cancerous), which are faster growing and can potentially spread to other parts of the brain or spine.

Tumours can arise in different parts of the brain and spinal cord, and symptoms depend on the area involved. Brain-tumour symptoms in children can be subtle or mimic more common illnesses, making early detection challenging. However, persistent or worsening symptoms should prompt medical review.

Common signs include:

- headaches, especially early in the morning or ones that wake a child from sleep
- nausea and vomiting, often alongside headaches and unrelated to food or illness
- balance and co-ordination issues, such as clumsiness, difficulty walking, or holding objects
- vision problems, such as blurred or double vision, squinting, or frequent eye complaints
- unusual eye movements or head tilting
- seizures, particularly if the child hasn't had them before
- personality or behavioural changes, such as unexplained irritability, drowsiness, or withdrawal
- developmental regression, such as losing previously gained skills, especially in young children

- growth or puberty changes caused by tumours near the pituitary gland, which can affect hormones.

Please note, however, that many of these symptoms are more likely caused by common childhood illnesses. However, if symptoms persist, are unexplained, or get worse, consult your GP.

How are brain tumours diagnosed?

If a brain tumour is suspected, your GP will refer your child to a specialist urgently, usually a paediatrician or paediatric neurologist.

Diagnostic steps include:

- a neurological examination to check reflexes, co-ordination, and function
- imaging tests, such as MRI or CT scans, which are the main tools used to detect a tumour's presence, location, and size
- further tests, including a biopsy if a tumour is found, to determine the type of tumour and guide treatment
- a lumbar puncture (spinal tap) is sometimes also needed.

In Ireland and the UK, children are seen through CHI or NHS specialist centres with access to multidisciplinary paediatric oncology teams.

What causes brain tumours in children?

Most childhood brain tumours develop without a clear cause. As we learn more through science and research, we may understand causes in years to come.

There is nothing a parent can do to prevent a brain tumour developing.

Prognosis and outlook

The outcome for childhood brain tumours varies widely. Some low-grade tumours can be cured with surgery alone, while high-grade or malignant tumours may require intensive treatment and carry a more guarded prognosis.

However, survival rates have improved significantly. For example, the five-year survival rate for some childhood brain tumours is now over 70%, but it depends on the tumour type and location.

Long-term follow-up is essential. Even after successful treatment, children may face challenges, and specialist support is available through neuro-oncology rehabilitation services, educational psychologists, and support charities.

WILMS TUMOUR

> ### FREDDIE'S STORY
> Aoife was giving three-year-old Freddie a bath when she felt a hard lump in his tummy. It felt very big, but it didn't hurt Freddie when she pressed on it. She was worried, so she brought Freddie to her GP, who was also able to feel the lump. The GP referred Freddie to the emergency department in the local hospital, where a scan of his tummy showed a large mass.

Wilms tumour, also known as nephroblastoma, is a rare type of kidney cancer that primarily affects children under the age of five. The exact cause is not known, but genetics are thought to play a role, as they can run in families. Though it can sound frightening, the outlook for most children diagnosed with Wilms tumour is very good with prompt treatment.

It is the most common kidney cancer in children, though it is still rare and affects around 85 children each year in the UK, and around eight children per year in Ireland. It usually affects only one kidney, but in about 5–10% of cases, both kidneys may be involved.

Early symptoms can be vague, but common signs include:

- abdominal swelling or a firm mass that is often painless (the swelling might be noticed during bathing or dressing)
- abdominal pain
- blood in the urine (haematuria) that may appear pink, red, or brown
- fever
- loss of appetite
- fatigue or lethargy
- high blood pressure.

Because these symptoms are not specific to Wilms tumour, it's crucial to seek medical advice for any persistent or unexplained signs in your child.

There is nothing a parent can do to prevent a Wilms tumour developing.

How is Wilms tumour diagnosed?

If a doctor suspects Wilms tumour, they may refer your child to a paediatric oncology centre for further testing, which may include:

- an ultrasound scan of the abdomen
- an MRI or CT scan to determine the size and spread
- blood and urine tests
- a chest X-ray or CT scan to check if the cancer has spread to the lungs

- a biopsy to take a small sample of tissue to confirm the diagnosis in some cases.

The tumour is then staged based on its size, whether it has spread, and how it responds to initial treatment. The 'stage' of a tumour (one to four) helps the medical team to decide on the best treatments for the individual child.

Prognosis and outlook

With early diagnosis and proper treatment, the survival rate for Wilms tumour exceeds 90%. Most children recover fully and lead normal, healthy lives after treatment. Long-term follow-up is essential to monitor for any late effects of treatment or recurrence.

NEUROBLASTOMA

> ### SAM'S STORY
> Four-year-old Sam had been limping on and off for a month, and was unusually tired. He wasn't eating as well as he usually did and was also losing weight. His mum, Helen, could not pinpoint exactly what was wrong, but she felt strongly that there was something serious going on. She spoke to her GP, who referred her to the local Paediatric Assessment Unit, and Sam was admitted to hospital for tests.

Neuroblastoma is a cancer that develops from immature nerve cells called neuroblasts, which are part of the sympathetic nervous system. This system controls involuntary functions, such as heart rate and blood pressure. Neuroblastoma usually starts in the adrenal glands (located above the kidneys), but it can also develop in nerve tissues along the spine, chest, abdomen, or neck.

It primarily affects infants and young children, often under five years of age. Symptoms vary depending on the tumour's size and location, but may include:

- a lump or swelling under the skin, often in the abdomen, neck, or chest
- pain in the affected area
- fatigue and general weakness
- fever without infection
- weight loss or poor appetite
- changes in bowel or bladder habits
- swelling around the eyes or dark circles
- limping or difficulty walking if the tumour affects bones or nerves
- high blood pressure (if adrenal glands are involved).

Because these symptoms can be vague or mistaken for common childhood illnesses, persistent or unexplained signs should always be checked by a GP.

What causes neuroblastoma?

The exact cause of neuroblastoma is not fully understood. It arises when immature nerve cells fail to develop properly and begin to multiply uncontrollably. While most cases occur sporadically without a family history, a small percentage may be linked to inherited genetic mutations.

Research continues into genetic and environmental factors, but no direct cause or prevention method has been confirmed.

There is nothing a parent can do to prevent neuroblastoma from developing.

How is neuroblastoma diagnosed?

If neuroblastoma is suspected, your child's doctor will arrange for tests in hospital, which may include:

- physical examination to check for lumps, swelling, or other signs
- imaging tests, such as X-ray, ultrasound, MRI or CT scans, to locate and assess the tumour
- urine tests to detect certain chemicals produced by neuroblastoma cells, such as catecholamines
- a biopsy to take a small sample of tumour tissue to confirm the diagnosis
- bone-marrow tests to see if cancer has spread to the bone marrow.

Specialist paediatric oncologists and radiologists usually co-ordinate these tests at hospitals with dedicated children's cancer services.

Prognosis and outlook

The outlook for children with neuroblastoma varies widely, depending on:

- the age of the child at diagnosis
- the stage and risk group of the tumour
- the genetic features of the cancer cells.

Some neuroblastomas can regress spontaneously or respond very well to treatment, especially in infants and low-risk cases. However, high-risk neuroblastomas require intensive treatment and have a more challenging prognosis.

With advances in treatment, survival rates have improved

considerably over the past decades, and ongoing research continues to enhance outcomes.

SEEKING HELP

If you have spent time reading this chapter, it possibly means you have a serious concern about your child's health, and having major concerns can be very stressful.

The best place to start is by making an appointment with your child's GP. However, if you are seriously concerned for your little one's health and feel it is an emergency, contact the out-of-hours GP service or bring your child to the nearest emergency department.

If you are unsure when to seek help, use the following table as a guide:

Situation	What to Do
Minor symptoms not improving	GP within a few days
Lumps, weight loss, night sweats	GP or urgent referral
First seizure, breathing problems	Call 999 or go to the ED
General feeling that something's wrong	Trust your gut: see your GP

CHAPTER 11
Fits, Faints, and Funny Turns

Little children can do things that look absolutely dramatic and scary, but that are not caused by anything serious and will not do them any harm. The types of episodes that put your hearts crossways as parents usually include strange or unusual movements, a sudden change in colour, or a loss of consciousness.

In this chapter, we'll take a look at benign neonatal sleep myoclonus (BNSM), breath-holding and reflex anoxic seizures, febrile seizures (convulsions), infant shuddering spells, and tics.

BENIGN NEONATAL SLEEP MYOCLONUS (BNSM)

BNSM is a condition seen in newborns and young infants that involves sudden, jerky movements or twitching, usually of the arms, legs, or whole body, but only during sleep. These movements can resemble seizures but, importantly, they are not a form of epilepsy and have no long-term health implications.

BNSM typically starts in the first few days to weeks after birth and usually resolves on its own by the age of six months, often much sooner. We don't have exact statistics on how many babies develop BNSM, but it is something that I see often in my paediatric neurology practice. BNSM often runs in families.

What does it look like?

The movements associated with BNSM can vary, but below are some common features:

- twitches or jerks of the limbs or body during sleep
- movements that stop immediately when the baby is awakened
- episodes that may be rhythmic or irregular, lasting seconds to minutes
- the baby appears completely well when awake, with normal feeding, growth, and responsiveness.

These episodes often occur during light sleep and never when the baby is awake.

What causes BNSM?

The exact cause isn't fully understood, but it's believed to be linked to the immature nervous system of newborns. As their brains and sleep cycles develop, these movements naturally subside.

It's also important to note that BNSM is not triggered by any underlying illness or brain abnormality.

How is BNSM diagnosed?

Most cases of BNSM can be diagnosed clinically, based on the description of symptoms and a physical exam. If your baby is otherwise healthy and the episodes stop when they wake up, a GP or paediatrician can usually make the diagnosis confidently.

In uncertain cases, a video recording of the movements during sleep can be extremely helpful for your doctor. Rarely, tests, such as an EEG (electroencephalogram) or sleep study, may be done to rule out seizures or other conditions if there are unusual features.

When should parents be concerned?

Although BNSM is harmless, it's completely natural to worry. You should consult your GP or public-health nurse if:

- the movements occur while the baby is awake
- your baby seems unresponsive, stiff, or floppy during or after the episode
- the jerks are asymmetric (only on one side)
- there are other signs of illness (fever, poor feeding, vomiting)
- the episodes are frequent and get worse over time.

In these cases, your doctor may refer you to a paediatric neurologist for further evaluation.

For most families, the biggest challenge with BNSM is the anxiety it causes. Many parents initially fear that their baby is having seizures. However, when BNSM is properly identified, no treatment is needed. It is a transient, harmless phenomenon of early infancy. While it can be startling to witness, it does not indicate any long-term problems and typically resolves within a few months.

BREATH-HOLDING SPELLS AND REFLEX ANOXIC SEIZURES

As a parent, witnessing your child suddenly stop breathing or collapse can be a frightening experience. Breath-holding spells and reflex anoxic seizures are two similar yet distinct conditions that may present in young children, typically between six months and six years of age. While usually benign, it's crucial to understand how to recognise these events, manage them safely, and know when to seek medical help.

Breath-holding spells

> ### LILY'S STORY
>
> Lily was a healthy, developmentally normal toddler with no significant medical history. Her mother reported that over the previous two months, Lily had several episodes where, following a tantrum or being told 'no', she would cry hard, and then seemed to be unable to take a breath. Her lips and face would turn blue, and she would become limp and lose consciousness for a few seconds. She would regain consciousness spontaneously, resume breathing, and be back to normal within a minute.
>
> There was no drowsiness or confusion afterwards. There were no jerking movements, incontinence, or tongue biting. The episodes were always triggered by frustration or anger. No similar events occurred when she was sleeping.
>
> Lily was referred by her GP for review by a paediatrician, who made the diagnosis of cyanotic BHS, based on the history given by her parents and the fact that Lily had a normal physical examination.

Breath-holding spells (BHS) are non-epileptic episodes where a child involuntarily stops breathing, usually in response to distress or frustration. There are two main types:

- Cyanotic BHS: This is the most common form. Triggered by emotional upset (crying, tantrums), the child stops breathing, turns blue (especially around the lips), and may briefly lose consciousness.
- Pallid BHS: Typically triggered by sudden pain or fear, the child turns very pale and may lose consciousness without

much crying beforehand. These are also known as reflex anoxic seizures.

Reflex anoxic seizures

> ### DANIEL'S STORY
>
> Daniel was playing at nursery when another child accidentally knocked into him, causing a minor bump to the back of his head. He stood up, then suddenly turned very pale, collapsed, and appeared to stop breathing. Within a few seconds, he began to stiffen and had brief jerking movements of his arms and legs lasting less than 15 seconds. He was unconscious for under a minute and regained full awareness quickly afterwards, though he was briefly tired and tearful.
>
> His parents noted that this was the second episode in the previous three months, both triggered by minor injuries or fright. There was no family history of epilepsy or heart disease, and Daniel had no other health issues and was meeting developmental milestones.
>
> Daniel was referred by his GP for review by a paediatrician, who made the diagnosis of RAS, based on the history given by his parents and the fact that Daniel had a normal physical examination.

Reflex anoxic seizures (RAS) are sudden, brief losses of consciousness caused by an excessive vagal nerve response, most often triggered by minor injury or shock (e.g. bumping the head, witnessing something frightening). The child's heart stops for a second or two, or slows dramatically, leading to collapse. Seizure-like jerking movements may follow, but these are not epileptic.

Feature	Breath-Holding Spell	Reflex Anoxic Seizure
Trigger	Emotion (crying, tantrum) or minor trauma	Sudden pain or fright (e.g. bump to head)
Colour change	Blue (cyanotic) or pale (pallid)	Very pale or grey
Duration	Seconds to 1 minute	Usually less than 1 minute
Loss of consciousness	Sometimes	Almost always
Jerking or stiffening	Occasionally	Common (mimicking a seizure)
Recovery	Rapid, with no confusion afterwards	Rapid, child may be tired but alert soon after

What to do if an episode occurs

Witnessing your child lose consciousness can be scary, so making note of and following these steps might help you navigate an episode should one occur:

- Stay calm. Although terrifying, these episodes are usually not dangerous.
- Lay the child on their side or back. Ensure safety by preventing falls and loosening tight clothing.
- Do not try to shake, slap, or perform mouth-to-mouth. Breathing usually resumes naturally within seconds.
- Monitor recovery. Most children recover quickly and completely within a minute.

Seek emergency care if:

- the child takes several minutes to recover
- the child has persistent abnormal breathing or colour
- you are unsure if it was a seizure or something more serious.

Who to contact

Get in touch with your GP or public-health nurse for an initial evaluation and referral to a paediatrician if needed.

If the episode is prolonged or if breathing does not resume promptly, call emergency services (999/112).

Your child requires urgent medical attention if:

- they have an event without clear triggers
- they experience prolonged unconsciousness or confusion afterwards
- there is a family history of epilepsy, cardiac issues, or sudden death
- they have seizure-like activity.

In these cases, further investigation (e.g. ECG, EEG, blood tests) may be warranted to rule out epilepsy or cardiac arrhythmias.

Prognosis and long-term management

Both BHS and RAS are typically benign and self-limiting (they resolve by themselves without medical intervention). Most children outgrow them by age five to six, though occasional episodes may occur into later childhood.

There is no specific treatment for BHS or RAS, but certain management strategies can make things easier for you and your child:

- Reassurance and education: Helping caregivers understand the condition can reduce anxiety.
- Avoiding known triggers where possible: Manage tantrums gently and avoid sudden distress.
- Behavioural support: This is useful for children with frequent emotional triggers.
- Iron supplementation: Studies have shown that low iron levels (even without anaemia) may increase the frequency of episodes. Supplementing your child's diet with iron can significantly reduce the occurrence of episodes in some children, but only do so with medical supervision.

Although alarming, breath-holding spells and reflex anoxic seizures are usually harmless and temporary. With the right support and information, parents can feel more confident in handling these episodes. If you are unsure or concerned, seek professional medical guidance, especially if symptoms are changing or increasing in frequency.

An excellent resource for parents is the STARS website: www.heartrhythmalliance.org/stars.

FEBRILE SEIZURES/FEBRILE CONVULSIONS

PAUL'S STORY

Sarah, a mum of two, was making toast when she heard a thud. She rushed over to find her 18-month-old son, Paul, on the floor, eyes rolled back, arms jerking rhythmically. He wasn't responsive. She screamed for her partner, who called 999.

By the time the ambulance arrived, the seizure had

> stopped. Paul was groggy but breathing. He'd spiked a temperature with a mild ear infection. What Sarah witnessed was a febrile convulsion. Frightening but, in most cases, not dangerous.

The terms 'febrile seizures' and 'febrile convulsions' are interchangeable. They are seizures triggered by a fever, usually in children aged six months to six years. They're surprisingly common, affecting around 1 in 20 children in this age group in Ireland and the UK.

They are typically linked to viral infections and occur not because the child's temperature is especially high, but because it rises quickly. This is an important point: it's not how high the temperature climbs but how fast that causes problems.

A typical febrile seizure often involves:

- loss of consciousness
- stiffness, followed by jerking in the arms and legs
- eye-rolling
- clenched jaw or drooling
- shallow or paused breathing.

The seizures usually last less than five minutes and, afterwards, your child may be sleepy, floppy, or confused. This is called the 'post-ictal phase'. The word 'ictal' means seizure, so this means the phase after the seizure.

Watching your child lose consciousness and convulse is very frightening. So, if you've been through it or are living with that fear, you have my full empathy.

If your child does have a febrile seizure, you can do the following:

- Stay calm (I know, easier said than done!).
- Lay them on their side in the recovery position (see the NHS website, under 'Recovery Position, First Aid' for guidelines on how to do this).
- Do not restrain them.
- Do not put anything in their mouth.
- Time the seizure.
- If the seizure lasts more than five minutes or if it's their first, call 999/112.
- When it's over, let them rest. Don't rush them to drink or eat.
- Get them assessed by a doctor afterwards, even if they seem well.

What causes febrile seizures?

Febrile seizures are usually caused by viral infections, such as the flu, roseola, or ear infections, but they can also occur if a child has a fever for any reason. Some children are just more prone to them, especially if there's a family history of febrile seizures.

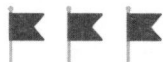

Always seek urgent care if:

- the seizure lasts more than five minutes
- your child is under six months or over six years old
- your child is not fully alert within 10–15 minutes
- the seizure affects only one side of your child's body
- your child has multiple seizures in 24 hours
- there is no clear source of fever.

Can you prevent febrile seizures?

This is important: you cannot reliably prevent febrile seizures.

Giving paracetamol or ibuprofen may make your child more comfortable, but it does not stop seizures from happening. Many parents are advised to treat every fever aggressively, but the science simply doesn't support that approach. So please, don't blame yourself for not 'catching' the fever quickly enough. You didn't do anything wrong.

Does having a febrile seizure mean my child will develop epilepsy?

Usually not. A simple febrile seizure (brief, generalised, and once in 24 hours) has a very low risk of progressing to epilepsy: about 2–4%, slightly higher than the general population.

The risk is a bit higher if:

- the seizures are long or focal (on one side of the body)
- your child has developmental delays
- there's a family history of epilepsy.

But most children do not develop epilepsy.

Prognosis and outlook

The outlook for children with febrile convulsions is usually excellent and most children outgrow them by age five or six. Most children affected will experience between one and three febrile convulsions in total.

There is no impact on your child's development, and they do not cause any lasting harm.

Febrile convulsions are scary to witness – when you've seen one, you don't forget it. But try to hold on to this: your child is almost certainly going to be absolutely fine.

And, for yourself, try not to carry the fear alone. Talk to your GP or other parents who've been there. We don't talk about febrile seizures enough but, when we do, we realise just how many of us have been through them.

INFANT SHUDDERING SPELLS

> ### OLIVIA'S STORY
>
> At around five months old, Olivia's mum noticed that she would occasionally stiffen her arms and give a quick shudder, like a goosebump reaction, especially during feeding or playtime. The episodes were sudden and lasted just a few seconds. Olivia didn't cry or seem distressed. In fact, she often smiled right afterwards.
>
> Worried it might be a seizure, her mum recorded a video on her phone and brought it to the GP. The doctor reviewed the footage and referred Olivia to a paediatric neurologist to be safe. An EEG and neurological exam were normal, and Olivia was diagnosed with benign shuddering attacks.
>
> Her mum was advised to continue monitoring the episodes and, by the time Olivia was 15 months old, they had completely disappeared. Olivia met all her developmental milestones and is now a thriving toddler.

If you've noticed your baby suddenly tremble or shiver without warning, you might be witnessing something called an 'infant shuddering spell'. Though they can look unsettling, these episodes are generally harmless.

Infant shuddering spells are brief, involuntary episodes that resemble a shiver or tremor. They can involve the head, neck, and shoulders, and may last only a second or two, though some may persist for up to 15 seconds. Your baby remains awake and alert throughout.

They may look similar to:

- a cold chill
- a startle response
- a seizure, which can be a concern at first glance.

Shuddering spells often begin between 6 and 12 months of age and typically resolve by two to three years old. They can occur multiple times a day or only occasionally.

What causes infant shuddering spells?

The cause is not fully understood, but the spells are believed to stem from immature neurological pathways in the developing brain. They are not caused by epilepsy, although they may resemble seizures to an untrained eye.

Triggers may include:

- feeding (especially when transitioning to solids)
- excitement or stimulation
- sudden body movement or a change in position.

How are infant shuddering spells diagnosed?

Diagnosis relies mainly on a clear history and, ideally, video evidence. Doctors will want to rule out:

- infantile spasms (a serious form of epilepsy)

- focal seizures (on just one side of the body or just one part of the body)
- movement disorders or metabolic issues.

If there's any doubt, an EEG (brain wave scan) or MRI may be recommended, though these are usually normal.

There is no treatment required for typical shuddering spells. However, to help diagnosis and monitor episodes, you can:

- record episodes on your phone to show your GP or paediatrician
- keep track of when and how often the spells happen
- ensure your baby is otherwise growing, feeding, and developing normally.

Seek medical advice from a GP or public-health nurse if:

- **your baby has spells during sleep**
- **there are changes in your baby's awareness, such as staring spells or loss of muscle tone**
- **your baby has a developmental delay or regression**
- **the episodes involve eye-rolling, jerking limbs, or your baby seems distressed afterwards.**

Prognosis and outlook

In otherwise healthy children, shuddering spells are not associated with developmental delays or neurological damage. Most children outgrow them completely within the first couple of years.

However, ongoing observation is important. Rarely, similar movements may be an early sign of:

- epileptic seizures, if accompanied by changes in awareness or development
- neurological disorders – particularly if developmental milestones are not being met.

Infant shuddering spells are usually benign. Though they may look strange, they rarely mean anything serious. Still, it's always wise to bring up any concerns with your GP or public-health nurse.

Appropriate monitoring and, if necessary, a neurological assessment reassures most parents, and most babies simply outgrow the spells as their nervous systems mature.

TICS

> ### EMMA'S STORY
> Emma, aged four, was a bright, playful child whose parents noticed she had begun blinking excessively and making a quiet grunting sound when she was playing. These behaviours seemed to come and go, sometimes disappearing for days. Concerned, her parents mentioned it to their GP, who observed the tics and referred her for a paediatric assessment. Emma was diagnosed with tic disorder, a condition that often resolves on its own. Her parents were reassured, and the paediatric team worked with them to reduce environmental stressors and monitor Emma's progress over time.

Tics can be a puzzling and sometimes worrying experience for parents of young children. They present as sudden, repetitive movements or sounds that your child makes involuntarily. While often harmless and temporary, understanding what tics are – and what they aren't – can help ease your concerns and guide you to seek support if needed.

Tics are sudden, rapid, repetitive movements or vocalisations that a person performs involuntarily. They are not deliberate and may become more noticeable when a child is excited, tired, stressed, or anxious.

There are two main types:

- Motor tics: These involve movements, such as blinking, facial grimacing, shoulder shrugging, or head jerking.
- Vocal tics: These include sounds, such as throat clearing, coughing, sniffing, grunting, or squeaking.

In young children, tics often appear intermittently and may come and go over time.

Tics usually begin between ages three and eight, often around age five. It's relatively uncommon to see tics before age two and, in these cases, a careful developmental review is advised to rule out other conditions.

What causes tics?

The exact cause of tics is not fully understood, but it's believed to be a mix of genetic, neurological, and environmental factors. Research shows that tics are linked to differences in how the brain processes movement and sensory information, particularly in the basal ganglia – structures deep within the brain that control movement.

Common tic triggers include:

- fatigue
- excitement
- stress or anxiety
- illness
- transitions (e.g. starting 'big school').

There is nothing a parent can do to prevent tics from developing.

How are tics diagnosed?

Tics are usually diagnosed based on clinical observation and history, often by a GP or paediatrician. Formal diagnosis does not usually require blood tests or brain scans, unless other neurological symptoms are present.

There are different diagnostic categories:

- Simple tic disorder: Tics that have been present for less than 12 months.
- Chronic motor- or vocal-tic disorder: Tics lasting more than 12 months, involving either motor or vocal tics.
- Tourette syndrome: When both motor and vocal tics are present for over 12 months.

Treatment options

For most young children, treatment isn't necessary, especially if the tics are mild and not disruptive. However, if intervention is needed, it may include:

- education for parents, as understanding tics reduces anxiety around them
- behavioural therapy – typically for older children
- support in educational settings, including awareness among teachers

- medications, though these are rarely used in very young children and are only for severe, impairing tics.

There are some things to keep in mind when coping with tics:

- Tics are common in early childhood and often temporary.
- They are not harmful and, in most cases, do not need treatment.
- Try not to draw attention to the tics or ask your child to stop.
- Seek support if tics persist, worsen, or are linked to other developmental concerns.
- A calm, supportive environment helps most children cope better.

Prognosis and outlook

The prognosis is generally good. Most children with tics will see improvement or complete resolution by adolescence. Around 1 in 10 may have more persistent symptoms into adulthood, especially if associated with other conditions.

In summary:

- Tics generally peak between ages 8 and 12
- They often become less frequent and severe with age
- Most children do not require treatment.

Are tics associated with other conditions?

Most children with tics do not have any other health or developmental issues. However, some children with tics may also have:

- ADHD (attention-deficit/hyperactivity disorder)
- autism spectrum condition

- obsessive-compulsive behaviours
- anxiety or sensory-processing differences.

It's important to note that not all children with tics have these conditions, and a full developmental assessment may be advised if there are wider concerns.

FINAL TIPS

When you are in the middle of witnessing something that looks scary or concerning, remember that your child's safety is the number one priority, and run these checks.

	More Reassuring (Usually Benign)	More Concerning (Needs Medical Attention)
Child's awareness	Alert before and after the episode; returns to baseline quickly	Unresponsive for a prolonged period; drowsy or confused long after the event
Breathing during event	Breathing normally before and after the event; brief pause with breath-holding spell only	Persistent breathing difficulty, noisy breathing, or no breathing at all
Skin colour	Brief pallor or blue colour that resolves within a minute (e.g. during breath-holding or RAS)	Pale, blue or grey colour lasting more than 1–2 minutes, especially with no recovery
Duration	Lasts less than 1 minute (breath-holding, reflex anoxic seizure, shudder) or under 5 minutes (febrile seizure)	Lasts more than 5 minutes; repeated episodes in a short time
Recovery	Quick return to normal behaviour, feeding, play, or interaction	Delayed recovery, prolonged sleepiness, vomiting, or limpness afterwards
Trigger	Obvious trigger: pain, fever, upset, sleep	No clear trigger, episode happened without warning

	More Reassuring (Usually Benign)	More Concerning (Needs Medical Attention)
Movements	Rhythmic jerks during sleep (BNSM); brief stiffening or shaking with known trigger; no movement at all	Repetitive jerking with loss of consciousness; asymmetrical movement or stiffness with no known reason
Frequency	Single event or rare; improving over time	Repeated or increasing episodes; happening more often or changing in pattern
Age	Fits expected pattern for age (e.g. BNSM in young baby; febrile seizure in toddler)	Unusual age for type of event (e.g. seizure-like episode in newborn with no fever)
Overall health	Child is well before and after episode; normal development	Delayed development, other signs of illness (e.g. high-pitched cry, poor feeding, ongoing fever)

CHAPTER 12

Hospital Visits and Doctors' Appointments

You might never need to bring your little one to hospital, but there will be doctors' appointments to deal with at various points in your child's life. It is always helpful to be prepared for these visits because, in the middle of a busy clinic, with your child getting bored or asking for snacks, it can be hard to remember all the questions you want to ask or all the information you receive.

In this chapter, you will find tips and tricks for dealing with every kind of medical appointment, from the unplanned trip to the emergency department to the long-awaited appointment with a specialist.

MY STORY (ONE OF MANY!)

The playdate was going great. My two little girls had trotted off happily with their friends, giving me and my friend a chance to sit down with a cuppa and have a good old chat. About five minutes in, we heard a thump, a pause, and then wailing from upstairs. I recognised it as one of mine, sighed, and went towards the cries.

As soon as I saw the blood I knew that the playdate

was over, and the next stop was the local emergency department (ED). Somehow, my four-year-old had tripped going up the stairs, her lip had collided with a sharp edge and promptly burst open. There was a deep gash running through her lip and down onto her chin. No doubt about it, this would need stitches.

Because I was not at home, I was not able to gather the usual bits – snacks, entertainment for her, a charger for my phone, drinks – so we arrived in the ED completely unprepared. Now, because she was bleeding a lot, we were triaged and seen very quickly. We were told that this would need plastic surgery under anaesthetic. I could see my daughter's little eyes widening in horror.

The next piece of information came as a mixed blessing. We could go home after the wound was cleaned and come back early the next morning, fasting and ready for surgery. I say it was a mixed blessing because it gave us time to go home, get a good night's sleep, and prepare for the next day, but it also gave us time to get increasingly nervous! It involved us all: my youngest who had the accident, my older girl who witnessed the fall and was upset about her baby sister, my husband, who was worried about his little girl, and me, nervous about what was to come the next day.

We watched some cartoons on YouTube about going to hospital. My daughter asked if there would be a needle, and I told her about 'freddies' – that the doctors would put a little plastic straw (IV cannula) in her hand and it might scratch a bit going in, but then it would be all bandaged up and wouldn't hurt anymore. She asked if going to sleep would be scary, and I told her that I would be right there with her, and that she would breathe in magic air that smelled like bubble-gum, and would drift off into a lovely nap so that the doctors and nurses could do their job without her wriggling around.

Before heading off the next morning, I made a number of assumptions that made the visit a bit more challenging. I assumed we would arrive and she would more or less go straight to surgery. I forgot that she wasn't the only little child in the area who may have injured herself in the previous 24 hours, and that there may be others ahead of her needing anaesthetic and surgery.

I had decided to fast in 'solidarity' with her, so I also arrived at the hospital with an empty tummy and no snacks. Because I was so focused on the surgery and the presumption that it was imminent, I brought no entertainment for me or her. All we had was my phone – and, guess what? I hadn't brought the charger. When I was told at 8 am that her slot was at about 10.30 am, my stomach lurched. I'm not sure if it was hunger or anxiety!

Basically, I made all the mistakes so you don't have to! The surgery was a complete success, but I could have made the whole experience more comfortable if I had remembered that hospitals deal with much bigger emergencies than the one my daughter was facing and that, although her surgery was important, she was not top of the list, and that not having a good breakfast myself was a really silly idea!

Hospital visits, whether planned or unexpected, are among the more challenging experiences you'll face as a parent. When your child is a toddler or preschooler, it adds another layer of complexity. At this age, children are old enough to sense that something unusual is happening, but not always able to understand what or why. How you prepare, both practically and emotionally, can make a huge difference to their experience – and yours.

Let's take a look at the different types of hospital visits you may encounter, both elective (planned) and emergency, along with tips on what to pack, how to talk to your child about it, and how to prepare for medical appointments with your GP or a specialist consultant. That way you will be far more prepared than I was when we had our first trip to the ED with one of our kids.

WHEN THE VISIT IS PLANNED: ELECTIVE PROCEDURES AND TESTS

A planned hospital visit gives you the chance to prepare. You might have known about the appointment for weeks or even months, giving you time to get information from your child's consultant or GP, arrange childcare for siblings, and think through the logistics of the day or overnight stay.

Equally important is how you prepare your child. Toddlers and preschoolers don't need long, detailed explanations, but they do need to know what's going on. Start with simple, reassuring language. You might say, 'We're going to the hospital so the doctor can help you feel better' or 'You'll have a little sleep at the hospital, and I'll be right there when you wake up.'

Avoid overpromising. Statements like 'It won't hurt' can backfire if your child ends up having a blood test or injection. Instead, emphasise that doctors and nurses are there to help and that you'll be close by the whole time.

Reading a picture book about hospitals or playing doctors at home can be a lovely way to reduce anxiety. There are resources available from Children's Health Ireland, the NHS, and children's charities with gentle explanations and illustrations.

As the day approaches, pack a bag that includes familiar

HOSPITAL VISITS AND DOCTORS' APPOINTMENTS | 271

comforts. A favourite teddy, blanket, or bedtime book can make a sterile hospital environment feel a little more like home. Choose soft, comfortable clothes – pyjamas or a loose tracksuit are perfect. If your child uses nappies or pull-ups, bring more than you would usually need. Even if they're toilet trained, hospital stays can be unsettling, and regressions are completely normal.

Don't forget things for yourself. Most hospitals encourage a parent to stay, but facilities can be basic. A phone charger, water bottle, snacks, a toothbrush, and a change of clothes can go a long way when you're focused on your little one. If you have hospital letters or a care plan, keep them at the top of your bag for easy access.

WHEN THE VISIT IS UNEXPECTED: EMERGENCIES

You cannot plan for an emergency, but you can prepare yourself mentally for how to manage one. When I realised that my little girl needed to go to the ED, my main thoughts were *I hope she's okay* and *I can't believe this has happened*. Even when I arrived in the ED, it all felt unreal, like I was watching a movie of me and her. Dissociating was probably my way of coping, but I felt very aware that I needed to be present for my little girl. It is truly hard to carry your own feelings (worry and guilt: the terrible two) and the feelings of your little one.

If your child needs to be taken to the ED or urgent care, things might feel chaotic. Try to stay calm, even if you're frightened. Your child will look to you for cues. Speak gently and clearly, even if you are in a rush.

If you have time before leaving home or waiting for an ambulance, grab any medical records (like vaccinations), any medications your child is on, and a comfort item like a dummy, toy, or small blanket. Pack nappies, wipes, a change of clothes, and a snack if you can. Even if you don't use everything, having them to hand helps you feel a little more in control.

In the hospital, be prepared to wait. Emergency departments prioritise cases by urgency, not arrival time, so it's possible you'll be there for several hours. Some hospitals have play therapists or children's nurses who can help distract and reassure young patients. If your child is well enough, quiet activities that include picture books, sticker pads, or a tablet with headphones can help pass the time.

You may need to answer questions from different doctors and nurses. Don't worry if you're flustered – it's okay to say, 'I don't know' or 'Let me think for a moment.' If you're offered a leaflet or aftercare instructions, take it home and read it again later when things are less overwhelming.

Here's a checklist that might come in handy if you have an unexpected trip to the hospital.

For Your Child	For Yourself
Comfortable clothes or pyjamas	Comfortable clothes
Spare underwear or nappies	Toiletries (toothbrush, toothpaste, deodorant, etc.), underwear
Favourite toy, teddy, blanket, or comfort item	Phone and charger
Books, stickers, or quiet toys	Snacks and water bottle
Tablet with headphones (optional)	A book, magazine, or something to pass the time
Dummy or bottle (if used)	Hospital paperwork or letters
Any regular medication	Notebook and pen
Sippy cup or beaker	Wallet with ID, change or card for parking
Snacks or special foods (if allowed)	Any medications you need for yourself
Personal child health records	Hair tie, glasses or contact lenses if worn
Change of clothes (especially if overnight)	A small blanket or scarf (wards can be chilly)
Nappy cream or moisturiser (if needed)	Moisturiser and a neck pillow (think of it like a long-haul flight)

PREPARING FOR A GP VISIT

Routine GP appointments may not seem like a big deal but, to a toddler, they can feel confusing or even scary. The more predictable you can make the experience, the better.

Before the appointment, think through what you want to say. Write down your child's symptoms and how long they've been happening, especially if it's a long-standing or more complex issue. If your child is on any medication or has known allergies, jot those down too.

Explain the visit to your child simply. You might say, 'We're going to see the doctor. They'll listen to your chest and maybe look in your ears' or 'You'll sit on my lap and we'll show the doctor your spots.'

Try not to rush. If possible, arrive with a few minutes to spare so you can settle your child and use the waiting time to chat or play. Some GP surgeries have children's books and toys, but it's always wise to bring something familiar from home.

When you're in the appointment, remember you're the expert on your child, even if you're unsure what's wrong. Don't be afraid to say, 'I've noticed this and I'm not sure if it's normal' or 'It's probably nothing, but it's been worrying me.' GPs are used to this and it's always better to speak up.

SEEING A CONSULTANT: SPECIALIST APPOINTMENTS

When your child is referred to a consultant, it usually means there's a specific concern that needs deeper investigation. These appointments may be at a hospital or private clinic, and they often involve longer discussions, tests, or assessments.

Try to prepare by reading any referral letters, emails, texts, and hospital information in advance. Make a list of your questions, especially things you want to clarify or follow up on – it's easy to forget when you're in the room.

Depending on the clinic, you may be seen promptly or have a significant wait. Bring things to entertain your child and something for yourself to read or write in. Don't be surprised if a nurse or junior doctor sees you first to take a medical history.

You might feel overwhelmed by the amount of information given at these visits, especially if your child is diagnosed with a condition or sent for further tests. It's okay to ask for the information you are given to be explained in plain language or for it to be repeated. You can also ask for a summary in writing. Some hospitals will send you a copy of the clinic letter automatically.

Even if the appointment doesn't involve treatment that day, it can still be a lot for your child. Afterwards, do something comforting or familiar: stop at the park, read a special book, or cuddle on the sofa with a favourite movie when you get home.

EMOTIONAL SUPPORT

Preparing your child for hospital or medical visits is about more than just packing a bag. It's about offering reassurance, modelling calm, and helping them feel secure, even if you are feeling anxious yourself.

No matter the setting – GP, ED, or hospital ward – your presence is what makes the biggest difference to your child. You don't need to have all the answers. Just being there, holding their hand, and explaining things as simply and truthfully as you can will help your child feel safe in unfamiliar surroundings.

And remember: it's okay to ask for help. Nurses, doctors, hospital play specialists, and even other parents in the waiting room are often more than happy to share support, advice, or simply a kind word. You're not alone.

CHAPTER 13
Teething and Teeth

I bet you'll be astonished when I tell you that the best time to take your baby to the dentist is within six months of their first tooth coming through. It seems like overkill, right? I mean, they probably have four teeth, maximum!

And yet, that is in fact what is recommended. It enables the dentist to check that your baby's teeth are properly formed and developing correctly. Your dentist can give you good advice on teething and check that you have a good dental-care regime for your little one. And it enables your baby to become familiar with the sights, sounds, and smells of the dental surgery from a very young age.

Speaking of teething, how is it going? Years ago, an old paediatrician professor told me that teething causes only one thing – teeth. He was very dismissive of the symptoms that are commonly attributed to teething, such as drooling, irritability, tummy upset, and poor sleep. I accepted his hypothesis ... until I had babies of my own! And then I realised that every baby experiences teething differently.

For some it is a breeze but, for others, it can cause pain, discomfort, and tummy upset. During teething, the salivary glands become more active, and this increased saliva can lead to drooling, and possibly cause a 'drool rash' around the mouth. Lots more saliva gets swallowed as well, and this can lead to watery stools and increased nappy rash in some babies. So, no, for many babies, teething does not just cause teeth, it causes some uncomfortable symptoms. My old professor was wrong!

Common teething signs include:

- increased drooling
- red or swollen gums
- irritability or restlessness
- chewing on fingers or toys
- slightly raised temperature (but not a fever).

Comfort measures include:

- gently rubbing gums with a clean finger or a cold teething ring
- offering chilled (not frozen) teething toys.

If needed, ask your GP or pharmacist about pain relief, such as sugar-free paracetamol or ibuprofen (age-appropriate and only when necessary).

Most babies start teething around six months, although anywhere from 4–12 months is completely normal. The first little visitors are usually the bottom front teeth. From there, teeth tend to arrive in pairs and, by around age three, your child will likely have their full set of 20 baby teeth.

FIRST TOOTH? TIME TO BRUSH

The moment that first tooth appears, it's time to start brushing. It may seem early, but decay can begin as soon as teeth erupt. In fact, dental decay is one of the most common chronic conditions of childhood in both Ireland and the UK. In England, 25% of children aged five have visible signs of tooth decay. In Ireland, the figure is around 30% of children aged five, and many young children require extractions under general anaesthetic in hospital.

WHY BABY TEETH MATTER

Some parents wonder, if they're going to fall out anyway, does it really matter? The answer is yes – it matters more than you might think. Baby teeth play a vital role in your child's early development. They:

- help with chewing and proper nutrition
- support clear speech development
- hold space for the adult teeth to come in correctly
- contribute to your child's self-confidence and smile.

When baby teeth are lost too early, especially due to decay, it can cause pain, infections, and difficulty eating, and can even lead to misalignment of the adult teeth that follow. In some cases, untreated decay can affect the adult teeth growing beneath.

Even more importantly, a painful mouth can make everyday life harder: poor sleep, difficulty concentrating, low appetite, and social anxiety are all more common in children with dental problems.

HOW TO BRUSH BABY TEETH

Here's what brushing should look like in the early years:

- From first tooth to age three: Use a tiny smear of fluoride toothpaste (at least 1,000 ppm fluoride).
- From age three to six: Increase to a pea-sized amount of toothpaste (with 1,350–1,500 ppm fluoride).
- Brush twice a day, especially before bed.
- Help your child brush until they're at least seven years old. They don't yet have the dexterity to do a thorough job.

You'll find the fluoride amount listed on the back of the tube, usually under 'active ingredients' ('ppm' is a unit of measurement that stands for 'parts per million').

One important detail that many parents miss is not to rinse with water after brushing. Spitting out the foam is enough. Not rinsing lets the fluoride stay on the teeth to keep protecting them.

Children under seven shouldn't use mouthwash because they may accidentally swallow it, which can be harmful. Their swallowing reflex isn't fully developed until this age, so ingestion is more likely. If a young child swallows too much fluoride from mouthwash, it can upset their stomach and cause nausea or vomiting. Over time, regularly swallowing excess fluoride may also lead to dental fluorosis, a condition where white or brown streaks or spots form on developing teeth.

CHOOSING THE RIGHT TOOTHPASTE AND TOOTHBRUSH

Standing in the supermarket aisle faced with rows of children's toothbrushes and toothpastes can feel oddly overwhelming. But don't worry, choosing the right tools doesn't have to be complicated.

Toothpaste

Fluoride is the key ingredient to look for; it helps strengthen tooth enamel and makes it more resistant to decay. Go for toothpastes with:

- clearly stated fluoride levels (not 'low fluoride' unless advised by a dentist)
- a mild flavour if your child dislikes mint.

Avoid 'training' toothpastes with no fluoride. They may taste nice, but they won't protect your child's teeth. Whitening or charcoal pastes are not suitable for children.

Children's toothpaste is often sweeter or fruit-flavoured to make brushing easier, but always check the fluoride content.

Toothbrush

Choose a toothbrush that fits comfortably in your child's mouth and has:

- a small head
- soft bristles
- a non-slip, chunky handle that's easy for small hands to grip (and for you to help guide).

Some toothbrushes come with flashing lights or timers, which can make brushing more fun for your little one. Electric toothbrushes are also fine for children over the age of three, provided they're used gently and still with your help.

Change the toothbrush every three months, or sooner if the bristles look worn or splayed.

The goal is to brush for two minutes, twice a day, which is easier said than done with a wriggly toddler! Try making brushing fun and effective by:

- playing a toothbrushing song or using a timer app
- letting them choose a special toothbrush or toothpaste
- brushing your own teeth alongside them as a model
- taking turns: you brush their teeth first, then let them 'have a go'.

You should brush or supervise brushing until at least age seven. Children don't have the fine motor control to clean every surface on their own until around that age.

EATING AND DRINKING FOR STRONG TEETH

Teeth don't just need brushing, they also need a good routine around food and drink. And it's not just *what* children eat, but *when*. Frequent snacking, especially on sugary foods, keeps acid levels high in the mouth and doesn't give the tooth enamel a chance to recover.

A few golden rules:

- Stick to three meals and two snacks per day.
- Give only milk or water between meals.
- Avoid juice and squash, even the ones that say 'no added sugar'.
- Try to avoid food and milk right before bed unless you brush again after.

Tooth-friendly snack choices include:

- cheese
- unsweetened yogurt
- fresh fruit (in moderation)
- raw veggie sticks
- wholegrain toast or crackers.

Not-so-great choices include:

- raisins and dried fruit (they stick to teeth)
- biscuits, cakes, and sweetened cereals
- fruit juices or smoothies (even natural sugars are still sugars to your teeth).

SPOTTING TROUBLE: SIGNS OF DECAY

Tooth decay isn't always obvious at first. Some signs to look out for include:

- chalky white spots near the gums
- brown or black marks on the teeth
- sensitivity when eating or brushing
- persistent bad breath.

If you're worried, even just a little, book a dental check-up. Early treatment can save a tooth and prevent pain or distress down the line. Don't wait until there's a problem to go. Regular check-ups help catch issues before they become emergencies. As your child gets older, and their permanent teeth grow in, you can talk to your dentist about fissure sealants. Fissure sealants are a safe, protective coating applied to the chewing surfaces of children's back teeth. They act like a shield, filling in the tiny grooves where food and bacteria can get trapped, which makes brushing easier and helps prevent cavities. The process is quick, painless, and can protect your child's teeth from decay for several years.

IF A TOOTH IS INJURED

Children are energetic explorers and accidents can happen. Knowing what to do in the moment can make all the difference.
If a baby tooth gets knocked out:

- Do not try to put it back in (there is a risk of choking and damaging the underlying adult tooth).
- Rinse your child's mouth with water.
- Apply a cold compress to reduce swelling.
- Call your dentist for advice.

If a permanent tooth is knocked out:

- Hold the tooth by the crown, not the root.
- If it is dirty, rinse it briefly with milk or saliva (your child's).

- Try to reinsert it gently or keep it in milk (or your child's saliva).
- Get to the dentist within 30 minutes.

For a chipped or broken tooth:

- Save any tooth fragments if you can.
- Rinse your child's mouth gently.
- Use a cold compress to reduce the swelling.
- Book an urgent dental visit.

Dental health plays a huge role in a child's overall health. Unfortunately, both of my children did develop dental problems and it caused them significant discomfort. There's a lot of guilt that comes along with realising your child has cavities – and I know this from personal experience!

If I had my time back, I would have brought them for their first dentist visit a lot earlier (I waited until they were around four), and I would have been a lot more aware that a diet that is very high in fruit (even too much fresh fruit, let alone raisins!) can be damaging to teeth. And the bottles of milk at bedtime? I would have cut those out by age one at the latest. It might have been tough in the short run, but it would have spared them the pain of dental decay. Allowing a child to fall asleep with a bottle of milk (or worse, juice) can lead to 'bottle caries' or 'baby bottle decay'. Milk sugars pool around the teeth during sleep and there's no saliva to wash them away.

I thought we were doing everything right by brushing twice a day and avoiding sugary snacks, but I was wrong! Hindsight is a wonderful thing. Hopefully by sharing this dental information and my experience with you, I will have given you some foresight – and you won't have the same regrets I do about my children's dental health.

CHAPTER 14
Skin and Rashes

When a rash suddenly appears on your baby or child, it can be alarming, and you may be worried that it is something serious.

If your child has eczema and the rash suddenly gets worse, you may be concerned that the skin has become infected. Let's talk about the typical rash of eczema and how to recognise if a skin infection is developing.

We'll also delve into common rashes that may develop even if your child has no prior history of rashes or skin problems.

A good online resource for identifying rashes is www.dermnetnz.org, but if you have any concerns whatsoever about your baby's or child's skin, you should speak to your GP.

ECZEMA AND ITS CARE

Atopic eczema is a chronic inflammatory skin condition that often starts in infancy. It causes dry, itchy, cracked, and sore skin, particularly in skin creases, cheeks, and the trunk. It's common in children with a family history of allergies, asthma, or hay fever.

To manage eczema, you can do the following:

- Use moisturisers generously and frequently to keep your child's skin hydrated.

- If prescribed, use topical steroids for flare-ups to reduce inflammation.
- Use lukewarm water with soap substitutes when bathing (ask your pharmacist for recommendations). Avoid perfumed products and bubble baths.
- Avoid triggers – common irritants include wool, dust mites, overheating, and certain soaps or detergents.
- Choose soft cotton clothes and avoid synthetic fabrics.

Children with eczema are more prone to skin infections because of the disrupted skin barrier. There are some infections common with eczema:

Bacterial infections
- Cause: Caused mainly by Staphylococcus aureus.
- Signs: Yellow crusts, oozing, swelling, pain.
- Treatment: Topical or oral antibiotics. Hygiene and regular emollients help reduce recurrence.

Eczema herpeticum
- Cause: Caused by the herpes simplex virus, which causes cold sores.
- Signs: Painful, rapidly spreading blisters, fever, and unwell appearance.
- Treatment: Requires immediate medical attention and antiviral medication.
- Note: This is a medical emergency.

Fungal infections
- Cause: Fungi, such as candida species.
- Signs: Round or oval red patches with a clearer centre, often with a more active, scaly edge. In darker skin, it may appear as darkened or lighter areas rather than red. It can mimic worsening eczema but may not respond to steroid creams and might even get worse with them.

- Common locations: Fungal infections can affect areas of eczema, especially in warm, moist parts of the body, such as groin folds (can be confused with nappy rash), between toes, under arms, on the scalp, under the neck, and behind the knees.
- Treatment: Topical antifungal creams (e.g. clotrimazole, miconazole). Oral antifungals may be needed if it is widespread or affecting the scalp.
- Note: Fungal infections may coexist with bacterial infections ('mixed infection') or be triggered by overuse of topical steroids.

INFECTIOUS RASHES IN CHILDREN

Many common infections in childhood cause rashes. Understanding how they spread and their risks is key, especially for pregnant women and those who are immunocompromised.

Meningitis and the non-blanching rash
- Cause: Bacterial meningitis (e.g. Neisseria meningitidis) or meningococcal septicaemia.
- Symptoms: High fever, vomiting, irritability, cold hands/feet, pale/blotchy skin, and a non-blanching rash (one that does not fade under pressure of a clear glass).
- Spread: Saliva, close prolonged contact.
- Treatment: Immediate hospitalisation and IV antibiotics. It is a time-critical condition.
- Pregnancy: No specific foetal risk but urgent care is always required for exposed household contacts.

Slapped cheek syndrome (fifth disease)
- Cause: Parvovirus B19.
- Symptoms: Flu-like symptoms followed by a bright-red rash on cheeks and lacy rash on limbs.

- Spread: Respiratory droplets. It is contagious before the rash appears.
- Treatment: Supportive – rest, fluids, paracetamol.
- Pregnancy: Expectant mothers who are non-immune to parvovirus can become infected. The virus can cross the placenta, which causes a risk of foetal anaemia, hydrops fetalis, or miscarriage, especially if exposed before 20 weeks. If you are exposed and pregnant, contact your GP or midwife urgently for monitoring (which may require blood tests or an ultrasound).

Hand, foot, and mouth disease
- Cause: Coxsackievirus A16 or enteroviruses.
- Symptoms: Fever, sore throat, painful mouth ulcers, and a rash with blisters on hands, feet, and buttocks.
- Spread: Contact with nasal secretions, saliva, fluid from blisters, and faeces.
- Treatment: Supportive – paracetamol/ibuprofen, fluids, soft food diet.
- Pregnancy: Generally low risk.

Roseola (sixth disease)
- Cause: Human herpesvirus 6 or 7.
- Symptoms: Sudden high fever, lasting three to five days, followed by a pink rash starting on the trunk, spreading to limbs.
- Spread: Saliva, often from older siblings.
- Treatment: Supportive – fluids, antipyretics (paracetamol or ibuprofen).
- Pregnancy: No known risk to unborn babies.

Scarlet fever
- Cause: Group A Streptococcus bacteria.
- Symptoms: Sore throat, fever, headache, red 'strawberry'

tongue, and a rough-feeling red rash starting on the chest/neck.
- Spread: Respiratory droplets and direct contact. Can return to school/childcare 24 hours after starting antibiotics.
- Treatment: Ten-day course of antibiotics (usually penicillin). Paracetamol for fever, plenty of fluids.
- Pregnancy: Generally mild in pregnancy but avoid close contact during infection.

Herpes simplex virus (cold sores)
- Cause: HSV-1 (oral); sometimes HSV-2.
- Symptoms: Small blisters around lips and mouth; in infants it can cause gingivostomatitis (painful gums, fever).
- Spread: Direct contact with saliva or sores.
- Treatment: Antiviral creams (e.g. aciclovir). For widespread or severe cases, oral antivirals may be needed.
- Eczema complication: In children with eczema, HSV can cause eczema herpeticum – this is a medical emergency.
- Pregnancy: The cold-sore virus (HSV-1) is not generally a problem for someone who is pregnant and has had cold sores before, as they will have immunity. If someone is pregnant and has never had cold sores and is exposed to a toddler with cold sores, careful handwashing and avoiding kissing an affected child on the mouth will help to reduce the chances of transmission.

Chickenpox (varicella)
- Cause: Varicella-zoster virus.
- Symptoms: Fever, fatigue, then a very itchy rash with red spots that blister and scab.
- Spread: Airborne droplets and direct contact. Infectious 1–2 days before rash appears until all blisters crust over.
- Treatment: Paracetamol (avoid ibuprofen), antihistamines, fluids. Calamine lotion or cooling gels may help.

- Pregnancy: Can be serious. Risk to the baby includes congenital varicella syndrome if infected early in pregnancy, or severe neonatal infection if contracted near birth. Contact your GP urgently if you are exposed and have never had chickenpox or the chickenpox vaccine, because this means you are not immune to chickenpox.

Measles
- Cause: Measles virus.
- Symptoms: Cough, conjunctivitis, high fever, white mouth spots (Koplik spots), then a spreading red rash.
- Spread: Extremely contagious via airborne droplets. Can live in air for up to two hours.
- Treatment: Supportive – fluids, rest, paracetamol. Hospital care if complications arise, e.g. pneumonia, encephalitis.
- Prevention: MMR vaccine (two doses).
- Pregnancy: High risk. Can cause miscarriage, premature labour, or stillbirth. Non-immune (never had measles or the measles vaccine) pregnant women who are exposed should seek urgent advice.

Impetigo
- Cause: Bacterial (staph or strep).
- Symptoms: Red sores that ooze then form golden-yellow crusts. Common around nose and mouth.
- Spread: Highly contagious via direct skin contact and contaminated items (e.g. towels and bedding). Exclude from school/childcare until 48 hours after starting treatment.
- Treatment: Antibiotic creams or oral antibiotics.
- Pregnancy: No known risk to unborn babies.

Ringworm (tinea)
- Cause: Fungal infection.
- Symptoms: Circular, red, scaly patches with a clear centre. Scalp ringworm may cause hair loss.
- Spread: Direct contact with infected skin, pets, shared

combs, or towels. No exclusion from school/childcare unless child has infected scalp or open sores.
- Treatment: Antifungal creams; oral antifungals for scalp involvement.
- Pregnancy: No known risk to unborn babies.

Molluscum contagiosum
- Cause: Poxvirus.
- Symptoms: Small, firm, dome-shaped bumps with central dimples. Common on body, limbs, and behind knees.
- Spread: Skin-to-skin contact, towels, swimming pools.
- Treatment: Usually self-resolves over 6–18 months. No treatment is needed unless the bumps become inflamed or infected. If you notice the bumps becoming red or developing pus, visit the GP.
- Pregnancy: Harmless in pregnancy.

Scabies
- Cause: Scabies is a type of infectious rash that has made a comeback in recent years. Unlike the infectious rashes listed previously, scabies is caused by a parasite. Many parents are aghast when their child is diagnosed with scabies, but it is important to remember that scabies is not a reflection of the hygiene practices in your home; it is caused by the Sarcoptes scabiei mite.
- Symptoms: Intense itching (especially at night), a bumpy, red rash with small burrow lines (thin, wavy grey or skin-coloured lines) often seen between the fingers, wrists, elbows, armpits, waistline, and, in young children, also on the face, scalp, palms, and soles of the feet. Infants may be generally irritable, and have difficulty sleeping.
- Spread: Spreads easily in households, schools, and nurseries through prolonged skin-to-skin contact or sharing of bedding and clothing. Children can return to school or crèche 24 hours after the first treatment.

290 | SHOULD I BE WORRIED?

Condition	Cause	Rash Description	Other Symptoms	How It Spreads	Treatment	Pregnancy Risk
Meningitis (bacterial)	N. meningitidis, others	Purplish, non-blanching rash (does not fade under pressure)	High fever, cold hands/feet, lethargy, stiff neck	Respiratory droplets, close contact	Emergency care, IV antibiotics	No direct foetal risk, but urgent action essential
Slapped cheek (fifth disease)	Parvovirus B19	Bright-red cheeks; lacy rash on limbs	Mild fever, cold-like symptoms	Respiratory droplets, contagious before rash appears	Supportive only	Significant risk: foetal anaemia, miscarriage – seek advice if exposed
Scarlet fever	Group A Streptococcus	Fine, sandpaper-like red rash starting on chest	Sore throat, strawberry tongue, fever	Respiratory droplets, direct contact	Oral antibiotics (penicillin), supportive care	Mild; avoid close contact if pregnant
Measles	Measles virus	Red, blotchy rash starting on face and behind ears	Fever, cough, conjunctivitis, Koplik spots	Airborne; extremely contagious	Supportive; isolation; prevent with MMR	High risk: miscarriage, stillbirth, premature birth
Chickenpox	Varicella-zoster virus	Red spots that blister, burst, and crust	Fever, irritability, tiredness	Airborne and contact	Supportive; antihistamines, calamine lotion	Risk of congenital infection; urgent advice needed
Hand, foot, and mouth	Coxsackie/enteroviruses	Small blisters on hands, feet, and mouth	Fever, sore throat, poor appetite	Saliva, nasal fluid, faeces	Supportive; fluids, soft foods	Low risk
Roseola	HHV-6 or HHV-7	Pink rash appears after fever; starts on torso	Sudden high fever, irritability	Saliva, especially from older children	Supportive; fever control	No known risk
Herpes simplex (cold sores)	HSV-1/HSV-2	Small clustered blisters, often around mouth	Painful gums (gingivostomatitis), fever in young children	Saliva, direct contact with sores	Antivirals (aciclovir); hygiene	Can be dangerous in newborns if primary infection
Impetigo	Staph or strep bacteria	Golden-crusted sores, often around nose and mouth	Mild fever (sometimes), local discomfort	Skin contact, contaminated items	Topical/oral antibiotics	No specific risk
Ringworm (tinea)	Fungal (various dermatophytes)	Ring-shaped, scaly red patches with a clearer centre	Itching, sometimes mild redness or cracking	Skin contact, pets, shared items	Antifungal creams/orals	No known risk
Molluscum contagiosum	Poxvirus	Small, dome-shaped bumps with central dimple	Usually none; can itch or become inflamed	Skin contact, towels, shared baths	Self-resolving (6–18 months)	Harmless in pregnancy

- Diagnosis: Diagnosis is usually made by your doctor based on appearance and history of exposure.
- Treatment: Application of a topical insecticide, such as permethrin cream, to the entire body (including the scalp in children under two). This should be repeated after seven days to kill newly hatched mites. All household members and close contacts should be treated simultaneously, even if they do not show any symptoms. Itching may persist for several weeks after treatment (a reaction to dead mites) and may require antihistamines or topical steroids for comfort.
- Pregnancy: No known risk to unborn babies.
- Note: Wash clothing, bedding, and towels at 60°C or above, or seal in a plastic bag for 72 hours. Scabies is not dangerous but is very uncomfortable and often under-recognised. Early treatment and treating all close contacts to the infected person are key to stopping its spread.

NON-INFECTIOUS RASHES IN CHILDREN

These rashes are not caused by infections and are not contagious, though they are often itchy and uncomfortable. They're often linked to allergens, sensitivities, or triggered by viral infections.

If your child develops an itchy or uncomfortable rash, they should be reviewed by their GP. A hive-like or red rash that develops suddenly can be a sign of a severe allergic reaction or anaphylaxis – in that situation, you should call 999/112.

Urticaria (hives)
- Cause: Allergies (foods, medications, insect stings), infections, or unknown triggers.

- Symptoms: Itchy, raised red or white welts, which often move around the body.
- Treatment: Your GP may advise antihistamines. You should also identify and avoid triggers.
- Emergency: Seek immediate help if breathing difficulty, facial swelling, or vomiting occur (anaphylaxis: call 999).

Eczema flare-ups from allergens
- Cause: Dust mites, pollen, animal dander, or food allergies.
- Symptoms: Increased redness, itchiness, or weeping in areas of chronic eczema.
- Treatment: Your GP may advise emollients, topical steroids, antihistamines. Allergy testing may be helpful.

Contact dermatitis
- Cause: Skin contact with allergens or irritants (e.g. nickel, soaps, cleaning products).
- Symptoms: Red, itchy, possibly blistered skin in contact areas.
- Treatment: Your GP may advise moisturisers and corticosteroid creams during flares. You should also identify and avoid triggers.

Psoriasis
- Cause: Immune system triggers rapid skin cell turnover, often influenced by infections, stress, skin injury or cold weather
- Symptoms: Red, scaly plaques on elbows, knees, scalp, or lower back. Itching, soreness, cracked or bleeding skin. Nail pitting and occasional joint pain or stiffness.
- Treatment: Emollients and prescribed topical therapies. Phototherapy for persistent cases. Systemic medicines for severe disease under paediatric dermatology care.

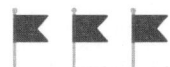

You should seek medical attention if:

- a rash is spreading quickly or looks infected (red, hot, weeping)
- your child has a high fever with a rash, especially a non-blanching rash
- there are signs of allergic reaction: swelling, breathing difficulty, facial rash
- your child is very unwell, drowsy, or hard to wake
- you're pregnant and have been exposed to measles, chickenpox, or slapped cheek.

Understanding the cause of a rash can bring peace of mind. Most are mild, short-lived, and treatable at home, but some need medical attention, especially when linked to infection, pregnancy risk, or allergic reaction.

Trust your instincts as a parent and, when in doubt, seek help.

CHAPTER 15
A to Z

Parenting has changed quite a bit over the past 20 years. With the advances in online search engines and social media, a lot of parents turn to their phone, tablet, or computer when looking for answers about their child's health. Although some of the information found online can be excellent and evidence based, unfortunately, some of it can be incorrect or misleading.

This chapter is an A–Z of the most-searched-for health conditions for babies and children from birth to five years old. Many of these conditions have been covered in earlier chapters and, where this is the case, there is a page reference so that you can refer back to those chapters for more details.

ADENOIDS

Adenoids are a small but important part of your child's immune system, especially in the early years of their life. Located high at the back of the throat behind the nose, adenoids help to trap bacteria and viruses that enter through the nose. However, in some children, they can become enlarged and cause a range of symptoms that affect breathing, sleeping, and overall well-being.

Adenoids are lymphatic tissue similar to tonsils, but while tonsils are visible at the back of the throat, adenoids are hidden behind the nasal cavity and can only be seen with special instruments. They are most active between birth and age five, and they typically begin to shrink after the age of seven, often disappearing by the teenage years.

Signs of enlarged adenoids

Enlarged adenoids can cause various symptoms, often mistaken for persistent colds or allergies. Here are some common signs to watch for:

- Mouth breathing: Your child may breathe mainly through the mouth, especially during sleep.
- Snoring or noisy breathing at night: Enlarged adenoids can block the nasal passages, leading to snoring or laboured breathing.
- Sleep disturbances: Children may experience restless sleep, pauses in breathing (sleep apnoea), or frequent waking.
- Nasal-sounding speech: Speech may sound muffled or as though the nose is constantly blocked.
- Persistent runny nose or nasal congestion: Even without a cold, the nose may seem constantly blocked.
- Recurrent ear infections or glue ear: Blocked Eustachian tubes due to enlarged adenoids can lead to fluid build-up and infections.
- Difficulty swallowing or a poor appetite: In severe cases, the enlarged tissue can make eating uncomfortable, which can lead to weight loss.

If you notice several of these symptoms lasting more than a few weeks, it's worth discussing it with your GP.

Why do adenoids become enlarged?

Adenoids can become enlarged due to:

- frequent respiratory infections that can cause inflammation
- allergic reactions that lead to chronic swelling
- genetic predisposition – some children naturally have larger adenoids or adenoids that are more prone to swelling.

How are enlarged adenoids diagnosed?

Your GP may refer your child to an ear, nose, and throat (ENT) specialist. Diagnosis typically involves:

- a physical examination
- an endoscopy, a small camera inserted through the nose
- imaging, such as X-rays
- hearing tests if ear issues are present.

Treatment options

The approach to treatment depends on the severity of the symptoms.

- Watchful waiting: If symptoms are mild, then no immediate treatment is needed. Many children outgrow the problem as their adenoids shrink naturally.
- Medication: For cases involving allergies or infection, nasal steroids or antihistamines may be prescribed to reduce inflammation.
- Surgery (adenoidectomy): If the adenoids are significantly affecting breathing, sleep, hearing, or causing recurrent ear infections, an adenoidectomy may be recommended. This is a short and commonly performed procedure, usually done under general anaesthetic as a day-case

surgery. Surgery is often combined with a tonsillectomy or the insertion of grommets (tiny tubes in the eardrum to relieve glue ear) if needed.

If you're concerned about your child's breathing, sleep, or hearing, don't hesitate to contact your GP for advice.

ALLERGIES

Allergies in young children often manifest as skin reactions, gastrointestinal discomfort, or respiratory symptoms. They can appear at any age, but many first emerge in infancy and early childhood.

Food allergies are often the earliest to be noticed, sometimes as soon as solid foods are introduced around six months of age.

Cow's-milk-protein allergy is one of the most common food allergies in infants. As children grow older, they may begin to show signs of environmental allergies, such as hay fever, triggered by pollen or dust mites. Asthma and eczema can also surface in the preschool or primary-school years, often linked to underlying allergic tendencies. In adolescence, new allergies may develop, including reactions to medications or insect stings, although many children also begin to grow out of some early food allergies during this period.

Recognising the symptoms

Allergy symptoms can vary widely, depending on the trigger and the child. In food allergies, you may notice hives, facial swelling, vomiting, or worsening eczema after your child has eaten certain foods. More serious reactions might include difficulty breathing, wheezing, or a drop in blood pressure, which might be signs of anaphylaxis – **this is a medical emergency**. (See pages 85 and 154 for more details on signs of anaphylaxis.)

Seasonal allergies, or hay fever, usually appear as sneezing, nasal congestion, itchy eyes, and a runny nose, often mistaken for a cold. Dust mites, pets, and mould can cause similar symptoms, especially indoors.

Insect stings and medication allergies may cause local swelling or hives but, in more sensitive children, they can also lead to systemic reactions, including anaphylaxis.

Getting a diagnosis

If you suspect your child has an allergy, the first step is to speak to your GP. They will review your child's medical history and symptoms, and they may refer you to a paediatric allergy clinic.

Diagnosis is based on a combination of clinical history and tests. Common investigations include skin-prick testing, where a tiny amount of allergen is applied to the skin to observe for a reaction, and specific IgE blood tests, which measure allergic antibodies in the bloodstream.

In more complex cases, an oral food challenge may be carried out under medical supervision, or an elimination diet might be tried, especially for suspected food allergies.

A clear diagnosis helps ensure that your child avoids unnecessary food restrictions or medications and receives the right treatment plan for their specific needs.

Managing allergies: short and long term

Management depends on the type and severity of the allergy. For mild symptoms, antihistamines can relieve itching, hives, or sneezing. Nasal sprays or eye drops may be used for environmental allergies, especially during pollen season. Moisturisers and steroid creams help with eczema flares.

For children at risk of severe allergic reactions, adrenaline auto-injectors, such as EpiPens or Jext pens, are prescribed. These should be carried at all times, along with an individualised allergy action plan, which outlines what to do in the event of an allergic reaction. Schools, nurseries, and caregivers should be trained in how to recognise symptoms and use the auto-injector if needed.

Avoidance of known triggers is essential. This might involve reading food labels carefully, creating allergen-safe environments, or managing pollen exposure through practical steps, such as closing windows during high-pollen days and washing hands and face after being outdoors.

In some cases, allergen immunotherapy may be recommended. This involves giving small, controlled doses of the allergen over time to build up tolerance, and is mainly used for pollen, dust-mite, or insect-sting allergies.

What to expect: outlook and prognosis

The long-term outlook for children with allergies varies. Many children outgrow certain food allergies, particularly to milk, egg, and wheat, by the time they start school. Allergies to peanuts, tree nuts, and seafood are more likely to persist into adulthood. Eczema, asthma, and hay fever can fluctuate, with symptoms improving or worsening over time.

Importantly, with the right management and support, most children with allergies live active, healthy lives. Ongoing follow-up with healthcare providers helps ensure that your child's treatment plan stays up to date and their needs are met as they grow. (See page 83 for more information about allergies.)

What about allergies to pollen or animals?

An allergy to pollen is called hayfever, and is covered on page 343.

You might notice that your child develops red, watery eyes or a skin rash when around certain animals. Common animals that children can be allergic to are cats, dogs, rabbits and horses.

Which is very unfortunate, because those are animals that many kids adore!

What causes animal allergies?
Animal allergies are usually triggered by tiny proteins found in:

- dander – flakes of skin shed by animals
- saliva – which gets on their fur when they lick themselves
- urine – especially in small pets like hamsters, mice, or rabbits.

These particles can float in the air, settle on furniture, and stick to clothes, which is why symptoms can appear even when the animal isn't nearby.

What are the symptoms?
Reactions vary from mild to more troublesome, and they can appear soon after contact. Signs include:

- sneezing, runny or blocked nose
- red, itchy, or watery eyes
- coughing or wheezing
- skin rashes or itching after touching an animal.

In children with asthma, animal allergies can sometimes make breathing symptoms worse.

How is it diagnosed?
If you suspect your child has an allergy, your GP may refer you to a specialist. Diagnosis usually involves:

- medical history – discussing when and where symptoms appear.
- skin-prick tests – a tiny amount of allergen is placed on the skin to see if there's a reaction.
- blood tests – which look for allergy-related antibodies.

How is it treated?
While there isn't a cure for pet allergies, the good news is that symptoms can usually be managed effectively. Many children find relief with medications such as antihistamines, which help ease sneezing and itching, or nasal sprays that reduce congestion. For those with asthma, inhalers can keep breathing symptoms under control. In some cases, older children or teenagers might be offered allergen immunotherapy, a long-term treatment that gradually helps the body become less sensitive to the allergen. With the right approach, most children can continue to live comfortably and enjoy being around animals.

The myth of the 'hypoallergenic' pet
You may have heard about 'hypoallergenic' cats or dogs – breeds that are said to cause fewer allergies. While some animals produce slightly less of the proteins that trigger reactions, no cat or dog is completely free of allergens. Even breeds marketed as hypoallergenic can still cause sneezing, itchy eyes, or asthma symptoms in sensitive children.

The key is not the breed, but how you manage exposure. Regular grooming, cleaning, and keeping pets out of bedrooms often have a much bigger impact on symptoms than the type of animal. In other words, loving your pet responsibly and taking a few practical steps can make life much easier for a child with allergies – regardless of breed.

What about keeping the family pet?
A diagnosis of a pet allergy doesn't automatically mean saying goodbye to a much-loved family member. Many families successfully manage allergies while keeping their cat, dog, or small pet. It often means making small adjustments: keeping pets out of bedrooms, washing hands and changing clothes after playtime, and using HEPA filters or vacuum cleaners to reduce dander in the home. Regular grooming and cleaning of cages or bedding can also make a big difference.

For some children, symptoms may be more severe, and if medical advice suggests it, finding a new home for the pet might need to be considered. But for most families, with thoughtful management and support from healthcare professionals, children and their pets can continue to share a happy, healthy home together.

BEDWETTING

Bedwetting (enuresis) is considered a normal part of development for many children up to the age of five or six. It is more common in boys than girls, and it tends to run in families – if one or both parents wet the bed as children, their own children are more likely to do the same.

Even at age seven, about 1 in 10 children still wet the bed occasionally. While frustrating, this is not unusual. Most children will outgrow it without needing medical treatment. However, you might want to consult your GP or a continence specialist if:

- your child is seven or older and continues to wet the bed regularly
- they were dry for six months or more and start wetting again (secondary enuresis)
- bedwetting is accompanied by daytime symptoms, such as frequent urination, urgent toilet needs, or accidents
- your child snores heavily, seems overly tired during the day, or has very large wet patches, which could suggest sleep apnoea or overproduction of urine at night.

Why does bedwetting happen?

It's important to know that bedwetting is not deliberate. Children are not being lazy or defiant. They do not wake because their brain hasn't yet developed the ability to respond to a full bladder during sleep.

This is because, as the brain matures, it starts to produce a hormone called antidiuretic hormone (ADH) at night. ADH reduces urine production during sleep. Some children's brains take longer to begin this nighttime hormone surge, meaning they produce too much urine while they are asleep and can't hold it all.

Other children may not yet recognise the body's internal signal to wake up when their bladder is full. This is not something they can control. It's a developmental issue, not a behavioural one.

Secondary bedwetting

If your child was dry, then starts wetting again, it's called secondary bedwetting (secondary enuresis). It can sometimes be triggered by:

- emotional stress, such as a house move, a new sibling, or school pressure
- constipation, which can put pressure on the bladder
- urinary tract infections (UTIs)
- sleep disorders
- diabetes, in rare cases.

If your child starts bedwetting again after a long dry period, speak to your GP to rule out medical causes or stressors.

When to seek medical review

You should consult your doctor if:

- your child is over seven years old and bedwetting persists
- bedwetting started suddenly after a long dry spell
- your child experiences pain or a burning feeling when they pee, or has blood in their urine

- there's a family history of diabetes, or your child is unusually thirsty, tired, or losing weight
- you feel overwhelmed or unsure how to help your child cope.

GPs can refer you to local paediatric specialists for support.

Management strategies

You can support your child at home with the following measures:

- Encouragement and reassurance: Never punish or shame. Praise dry nights, but don't criticise wet ones.
- Good toilet habits: Encourage regular toilet visits during the day and before bed.
- Avoid drinks with caffeine or artificial sweeteners.
- Fluid intake: Ensure your child drinks plenty during the day, but reduce fluid intake in the hour before bedtime.
- Nighttime routine: Use absorbent bed pads or protective covers, and make changes easy. Keep spare pyjamas and bedding nearby.
- Bedwetting alarms: These can help train the brain to wake up when the bladder is full, but they take time and consistency.
- Medication: If needed, a doctor may prescribe desmopressin, which mimics ADH and reduces urine production overnight. This is often used short-term for camps or holidays.

What's the prognosis?

The good news is that most children outgrow bedwetting. It may take time, and some may need extra support, but long-term issues are rare.

By the teenage years, fewer than 1 in 100 still wet the bed regularly. The key is patience, compassion, and a proactive approach.

BREATHING PROBLEMS

Children under two years

Young babies and toddlers have small, easily blocked airways. Even mild infections can mean they have trouble breathing. Common causes include:

- Bronchiolitis: A viral infection (often RSV, see page 98) that inflames the small airways. It is most common in babies under one.
- Reactive airways: Inflammation and a narrowing of the airways in response to viruses or irritants. It is sometimes a precursor to asthma.
- Bacterial pneumonia: A more serious infection with fever, chest congestion, and laboured breathing.

Children over two years

As children grow, they can describe symptoms more clearly, but breathing issues still need careful attention. Common causes include:

- Asthma: A long-term condition where airways narrow due to inflammation and muscle tightening. Often triggered by colds, allergens, or exercise. (See also page 185).
- Reactive airways: This is similar to asthma, but is triggered by infection.
- Bacterial pneumonia: This can cause fast breathing, chest pain, and a persistent cough.

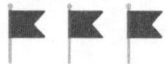

The red flags listed below mean your child may be seriously unwell and needs emergency care. If you notice any of these red flags, act immediately.

Red flags in children under two:

- fast breathing (see guide on page 307)
- nostrils flaring with each breath
- chest sucking in at the ribs or under the breastbone (chest recession)
- grunting noise when breathing out
- blue-tinged skin, lips, or tongue
- feeding less than half of their normal intake or refusing feeds
- drowsy, floppy, and difficult to wake
- pauses in breathing (apnoeas).

Red flags in children over two years:

- breathing rate faster than normal (see page 307)
- wheezing that doesn't improve with prescribed inhalers
- struggling to talk, eat, or drink due to breathlessness
- chest, tummy, or neck muscles visibly working harder to breathe
- blue lips, tongue, or skin
- unusually tired or drowsy
- fever with fast breathing and signs of chest pain or discomfort.

How to count your child's breathing rate

You don't need special equipment to count your child's breathing rate. All you need is a watch or timer, then you can do the following:

- Make sure your child is calm and not crying.
- Lay them flat or let them rest quietly.
- Watch the rise and fall of their chest or tummy.
- Count how many times they breathe in one minute (a breath = one rise and fall of their chest or tummy).

Age	Normal Rate (Breaths per minute)	Red Flag: Too Fast
Under 1 year	30–60	Over 60
1–2 years	25–40	Over 50
2–5 years	20–30	Over 40
5–12 years	16–24	Over 30
Over 12 years	12–20	Over 25

If your child is at rest and breathing faster than these limits, even without other signs, *get medical help*.

If your child has a cold and seems a bit off, it's usually okay to monitor them – but red-flag signs are not for waiting and watching. You don't need to know what's wrong, you just need to know what looks wrong.

If your child seems seriously unwell or their breathing is not right, get medical help straightaway.

CHICKENPOX

Chickenpox has an incubation period of 10–21 days, with most children developing symptoms about two weeks after they have been exposed to the virus.

Children become contagious one to two days before the rash

appears and remain so until all blisters have crusted over (usually five to seven days after the rash onset). This means they can spread the virus before you realise they have it.

Symptoms typically begin with:

- fever
- fatigue and irritability
- loss of appetite
- headache.

This is followed by the hallmark itchy, blister-like rash, which:

- starts on the chest, back, or face before spreading
- progresses from red spots to fluid-filled blisters that then scab over
- can number from a few dozen to several hundred.

While the illness usually resolves in 7–10 days, discomfort from itching and fever can be significant.

Chickenpox is contagious until all the spots have crusted over, so your child should stay at home and away from non-immune pregnant women, newborns, and anyone with a weakened immune system. (See the red flags on page 309 for more information.)

Treatment

If your child has uncomplicated chickenpox, the focus at home is on easing discomfort and preventing infection of the spots. Keep your child comfortable in loose, soft clothing and encourage plenty of rest and fluids. To reduce itching, you can use soothing baths containing oatmeal or bicarbonate of soda, apply calamine lotion, or give an age-appropriate antihistamine (check with your pharmacist or GP first).

Paracetamol can help with fever and aches, but avoid ibuprofen unless advised by a doctor, as it can increase the risk of skin complications.

Keep your child's nails short and clean to reduce scratching, and gently distract younger children with quiet play.

Potential complications

Though generally mild, chickenpox can cause serious complications, especially in:

- infants
- pregnant women
- people with weakened immune systems.

Complications include:

- skin infections
- pneumonia
- encephalitis (brain inflammation)
- sepsis.

Secondary infections from group A Streptococcus (strep A) are a rare but serious complication.

Contact a GP or seek urgent care if your child:

- has a high fever lasting more than four days
- is very drowsy or unresponsive
- has difficulty breathing or is fast breathing
- shows signs of a skin infection (red, hot, swollen areas, or pus filling the spots or oozing from the spots)
- has a severe headache, neck stiffness, or vomiting
- develops bleeding rashes or bruises.

In newborns or immunocompromised children, chickenpox should always be evaluated by a healthcare professional.

Vaccination

While the chickenpox vaccine has long been used in countries such as the US, it has not been routinely offered in Ireland. As of autumn 2025, the varicella vaccine has been added to the national childhood immunisation schedule.

Chickenpox is often seen as a 'rite of passage', but the discomfort and potential complications shouldn't be underestimated. With the rollout of the vaccine in Ireland, parents now have a highly effective way to prevent it.

CHOKING

We looked at choking in Chapter 5 (see pages 119–120), but it is something that really worries parents, so let's go over it again.

There are certain foods that the HSE and the NHS advise children under the age of five should not be given. This is because they pose a significant risk of choking.

These foods are:

- whole or chopped nuts (including peanuts)
- marshmallows
- popcorn
- chewing gum
- small, hard, round, or oval-shaped sweets
- small, hard chocolates.

Other foods require extra precaution when feeding to children under five:

- Small fruits and vegetables. Grapes and cherry tomatoes should be cut into quarters.
- Hard fruit and vegetables, such as carrots and apples. These should be grated or finely chopped.

- Food and fruit with skins, such as sausages, hot dogs, apples, pears, and tomatoes. These should be peeled and finely chopped.

Despite all the precautions you take, you may find yourself in a situation where your baby or child is choking. And remember – they can choke on small objects and toys as well as food.

I strongly advise you take a first-aid course and refresh your training regularly. This will give you the skills to deal with choking and other emergencies.

Signs your child is choking

A child who is truly choking will:

- be unable to cough, cry, speak, or breathe
- have silent, ineffective coughing
- show signs of distress or panic
- grab at their throat
- have blue-tinged skin or lips.

If the child is coughing forcefully or talking, encourage them to keep coughing – this means they still have some airflow.

First-aid guidelines for babies and children who are choking

For babies under age one
If you suspect your baby is choking and they cannot breathe or make noise, follow these first aid steps immediately.

Step 1: Check their mouth

Only if you can clearly see the object at the front of the mouth and can easily remove it with your fingers should you do so. Do not attempt to blindly sweep their mouth with your finger, as this can push the object deeper.

Step 2: Give five back blows

- Lay your baby face down along your forearm, supporting their head and jaw.
- Position their body so it is angled down towards the floor.
- Use the heel of your hand to give five sharp, firm back blows between the shoulder blades.

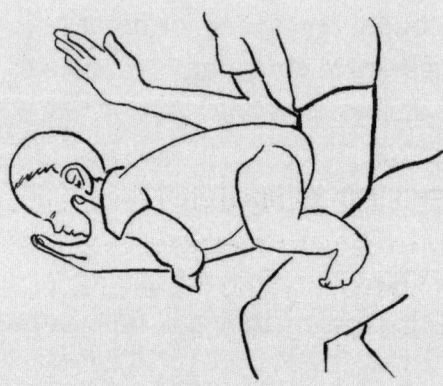

Back Blows

Step 3: Give five chest thrusts

- Turn your baby face up, resting them on your thigh or forearm.
- Place two fingers just below the nipple line, in the centre of the chest.

- Push inwards and upwards firmly but gently five times.
- Continue alternating five back blows and five chest thrusts until the object is expelled or help arrives.

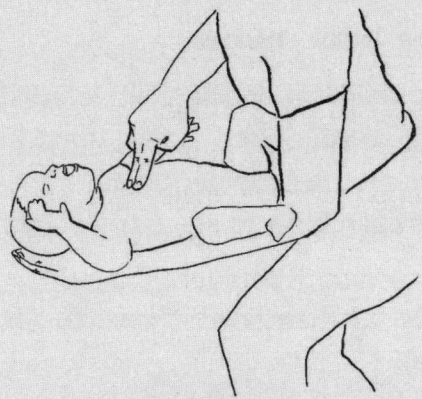

Chest Thrusts

If you have not already called the emergency services and your baby becomes unresponsive at any point, call 999/112 immediately and begin CPR (see pages 315–316).

For children over age one

Step 1: Check the situation

- Ask 'Are you choking?' If the child can speak or cough, do not perform back blows yet. Encourage coughing.
- If they can't respond or are making no sound, proceed to step 2 immediately.

- **Step 2: Call for help**
- Shout for help. If someone else is around, ask them to call 999/112.
- If you're alone, deliver first aid for up to one minute before calling emergency services.

Step 3: Give back blows

- Support the child by bending them forward at the waist.
- Use the heel of your hand to give up to five firm back blows between the shoulder blades.
- Check after each blow to see if the object is cleared.

Step 4: Give abdominal thrusts (Heimlich manoeuvre)

- Stand behind the child and wrap your arms around their waist.
- Make a fist with one hand and place it just above their belly button.
- Grasp your fist with the other hand and pull sharply inwards and upwards.
- Give up to five abdominal thrusts.
- Alternate between five back blows and five abdominal thrusts. Repeat this cycle until the object is expelled or the child becomes unresponsive.

If the child becomes unresponsive:

- Shout for help (if you haven't already).
- Call 999/112 immediately or send someone else to do so.
- Start CPR: begin chest compressions (30 compressions followed by 2 rescue breaths).

- Continue until emergency services arrive or the child recovers.

Even if the object is dislodged, always seek medical attention afterwards. The child may have internal injuries or residual obstruction.

CPR FOR BABIES, TODDLERS AND CHILDREN:

This guide is only an outline. It's not a substitute for hands-on training. To give CPR safely and effectively, parents should complete a certified paediatric first aid course – in Ireland, organisations like the Irish Red Cross, St John Ambulance, and the Order of Malta offer excellent training.

Still, it helps to know the basics in case of an emergency while waiting for professional help.

CPR for Babies (under 12 months)

Check responsiveness and breathing. Gently tap the baby's foot and call their name. If they're not breathing normally, call 999/112 immediately.

- Give rescue breaths. Cover both the baby's nose and mouth with your mouth and give 5 gentle puffs of air (just enough to see the chest rise).
- Chest compressions. Use two fingers in the centre of the chest, just below the nipple line (an imaginary line drawn across the chest from one nipple to the other). Press down about 4 cm (one-third the depth of the chest), 30 times at a steady rhythm.

- Cycle. Continue with 30 compressions and 2 breaths until help arrives.

CPR for Toddlers (1–5 years)

- Check responsiveness and breathing. If the child isn't breathing normally, shout for help and call 999/112.
- Rescue breaths. Seal your mouth over theirs (pinching the nose if possible) and give 5 gentle breaths, watching for chest rise.
- Chest compressions. Use one hand on the centre of the chest. Press down about 5 cm (one-third of chest depth), 30 times.
- Cycle. Continue with 30 compressions and 2 breaths.

CPR for Older Children (5+ years)

- Check responsiveness and breathing. Call 999/112 straight away if they are unresponsive and not breathing normally.
- Rescue breaths. Give 5 full breaths.
- Chest compressions. Use two hands, one on top of the other, pressing down firmly in the centre of the chest about 5 cm deep, 30 times.
- Cycle. Continue with 30 compressions and 2 breaths until emergency help takes over.

Final points:

- Always call 999 (or 112) if a child is unresponsive and not breathing. Place the call on speaker phone so your hands are free.
- If you're alone with a baby or toddler, and do not have a phone, do one minute of CPR before leaving to call for help. If they are small enough to carry, bring them with you to the phone.

- Even imperfect CPR is better than doing nothing.
- Most importantly: take a certified paediatric first aid course. Practising on a manikin with a trained instructor makes all the difference when you need to act under pressure.

COLIC

Colic is defined as episodes of intense, unexplained crying in an otherwise healthy and well-fed baby. Colic is something I experienced with my own baby, so I understand how incredibly tough it is. You can read my story on page 60 in Chapter 2.

The classic definition of colic involves crying for more than three hours a day, more than three days a week, for more than three weeks. It usually begins at around two or three weeks of age, peaks around six to seven weeks, and resolves by about three to four months.

These crying episodes often occur in the late afternoon or evening, and may be accompanied by clenched fists, an arched back, a red face, or pulling up of the legs. Despite how it looks, colic is not typically a sign of pain or illness.

What causes colic?

The cause of colic isn't fully understood, but there are several theories:

- Immature digestive system: Gas, trapped wind, or bowel spasms may contribute.
- Overstimulation: Newborns may struggle to filter out all the sensory input of their environment.
- Feeding issues: Swallowing air or reactions to cow's-milk protein may sometimes play a role.
- Normal developmental crying: Crying naturally increases in the early months of life.

SHOULD I BE WORRIED?

Importantly, colic is not your fault, and it doesn't mean your baby is unwell or that you're doing something wrong.

What is PURPLE crying?

You may come across the term 'PURPLE crying', which is used to describe the normal developmental stage where babies cry more than any other time in their lives. It's not a diagnosis, but a way to help parents understand this challenging phase. The letters stand for the following:

- **P**eak of crying: Crying increases around six weeks and improves after three to four months.
- **U**nexpected: Crying can start and stop for no clear reason.
- **R**esists soothing: Your baby may not calm down, no matter what you try.
- **P**ain-like face: Your baby may look like they're in pain, even if they're not.
- **L**ong-lasting: Crying spells may last for hours.
- **E**vening: Crying often happens in the late afternoon or evening.

Understanding that this is a normal, temporary stage can help reduce worry and guilt.

How is colic treated?

There is no single treatment that works for every baby, but some strategies may help ease symptoms:

- Try gentle soothing techniques: Swaddling, rocking, white noise, or using a sling or baby carrier.
- Burp frequently: Especially during and after feeds to help reduce trapped wind.
- Check feeding: Ensure a good latch if breastfeeding, or try a slower-flow teat for bottle feeding.
- Trial diet changes (under medical supervision): If breastfeeding, consider eliminating dairy for one to two weeks (under medical advice). Formula-fed babies might benefit from a hypoallergenic formula trial, as prescribed by a doctor.
- Create a calm environment: Dim lights, reduce noise, and avoid overstimulation.

Some parents find probiotic drops (particularly Lactobacillus reuteri) helpful in breastfed babies, but results are mixed and it may not help every baby. Simethicone drops are safe but have not shown clear benefits in studies.

Reflux medications are not recommended unless your baby has confirmed reflux disease.

What about chiropractors or osteopaths?

Gentle manual therapy is sometimes offered by chiropractors or osteopaths, and is often promoted as a treatment for colic. But the evidence is limited and inconsistent:

- A few small studies suggest modest improvements in crying time, but results are hard to interpret and haven't been widely replicated.
- There is no strong scientific consensus that these therapies work for colic.
- While rare, there are case reports of harm (especially with spinal manipulation in young infants).

The NHS and HSE do *not* recommend chiropractic care for babies because there is insufficient evidence and concerns about safety. Always consult your GP or paediatrician before considering alternative therapies.

While colic and PURPLE crying are usually harmless, certain signs may suggest something else is going on. Seek urgent medical attention if your baby:

- has a fever (above 38°C in a baby under three months)
- is not feeding well or is losing weight
- has projectile vomiting or green vomit
- passes blood in the stool or has very pale poo
- seems unusually sleepy, floppy, or unresponsive
- has a high-pitched or different-sounding cry.

Always trust your instincts. If something feels wrong, don't hesitate to get help.

The toll on parents: looking after your mental health

Caring for a crying baby who won't settle, day after day, is exhausting and distressing. Many parents report feeling anxious, overwhelmed, or even angry, and then feel guilty for having these feelings. This is completely normal. You are not alone, and you do not have to cope on your own.

If you are struggling, please talk to your:

- GP or GP practice nurse
- midwife or public-health nurse
- perinatal mental-health team, if available in your area.

You can also reach out to:

- Parentline Ireland
- Cry-sis Helpline (UK, for parents of babies who cry excessively)
- Samaritans (UK & Ireland)
- Local parent support groups, postnatal classes, or breastfeeding meet-ups.

If the crying becomes too much and you feel you might harm your baby:

- put your baby in their cot, somewhere safe, and walk away for a few minutes
- take deep breaths, phone a trusted friend, your partner, or a helpline
- never shake your baby, even briefly – shaking can cause serious, permanent brain damage.

If you feel overwhelmed or unsafe, go to the emergency department or call 999/112. Asking for help is a brave and responsible thing to do.

Outlook

Colic and PURPLE crying are incredibly difficult phases of early parenthood, but they are temporary. While there's no one-size-fits-all cure, there are ways to soothe your baby and protect your mental health. If you're feeling lost, remember: this stage will pass, and you are doing better than you think. Support is available; you don't have to carry this alone.

CROUP

Croup is a viral respiratory infection that causes inflammation and swelling in the upper airway, particularly around the voice box (larynx), windpipe (trachea), and the bronchi. It's most common in children aged six months to three years, though older children can also be affected.

Signs and symptoms

Croup often begins like a regular cold but quickly develops into more distinctive symptoms:

- Barking cough: A harsh, seal-like cough that is often worse at night.
- Hoarse voice: Due to inflammation of the vocal cords.
- Stridor: A high-pitched, noisy breathing sound when inhaling, especially when the child is agitated or crying.
- Mild fever: Usually less than 38.5°C.
- Laboured breathing: In more severe cases, breathing may become visibly difficult, with the child sucking in at the ribs or neck.

What causes croup?

Croup is usually caused by a viral infection, most commonly the parainfluenza virus. It spreads through droplets from coughs and sneezes, and it is most prevalent in the autumn and winter months. Children can catch it in crèches, schools, or from siblings.

Treatment at home

In most cases, croup is mild and can be safely managed at home. The key steps are:

- Keep calm: A child who is crying or distressed will often have worsened symptoms. Reassure them and hold them upright on your lap.
- Cold-air exposure: Taking your child outside into the cool night air or near an open freezer can help relieve symptoms. A 2023 observational study in *Pediatrics* found that cold outdoor-air exposure led to significant improvement in stridor and respiratory distress in children with mild croup. This supports the long-standing anecdotal practice many parents are familiar with.
- Hydration: Encourage small, frequent sips of water or diluted juice to keep your child well hydrated.
- Warm shower steam: Sitting in a steamy bathroom may help. Let a hot shower run with the bathroom door closed and sit nearby with your child. *Avoid steaming over bowls or kettles, as these pose a serious burn risk, especially for younger children.*

Medical treatment

If symptoms worsen or don't improve with home care, medical treatment may be necessary. Treatment, at your GP or in hospital, may include:

- Steroids: A single dose of oral dexamethasone or prednisolone is often prescribed. These reduce airway inflammation and have been proven to shorten the duration and severity of symptoms. Evidence shows that even a single dose improves symptoms within six hours and reduces the need for hospital admission.
- Nebulised adrenaline: Used in more severe cases to rapidly reduce swelling.
- Oxygen: If the child is having significant trouble breathing.

Call your GP, out-of-hours service or go to the ED if your child shows any of the following signs:

- **stridor at rest:** noisy breathing, even when calm and not crying
- **severe breathing difficulty:** chest retractions, flaring nostrils, or rapid breathing
- **blueness around lips or face:** a sign of low oxygen
- **drooling or trouble swallowing:** may suggest a more serious condition like epiglottitis
- **lethargy or unresponsiveness:** indicates severe illness
- **persistent or high fever:** particularly if accompanied by a rash.

Croup can be distressing for both child and parent, but with the right knowledge, most cases can be managed safely at home. Keep your child calm, stay alert for red flags, and don't hesitate to seek help if needed.

DEVELOPMENTAL DELAYS

Developmental milestones are skills or behaviours that most children can do by a certain age, such as sitting up, walking, or saying their first words. These markers help healthcare professionals monitor how children are developing physically, socially, and cognitively. They're useful tools, they are not diagnostic labels or parental report cards.

They are also *not* a race. There is a broad range of what is considered 'normal', and children can reach different milestones at different times. For example, some babies walk at nine months; others wait until 18 months. Both can be perfectly healthy.

When might a delay be a concern?

While variation is normal, it's also important to recognise when a child might be falling significantly behind in one or more areas. Developmental delays can appear in various domains, which we will go through now.

Gross-motor delays

Gross motor skills involve large muscle movements, such as crawling, standing, or walking. Signs to watch for:

- not sitting independently by nine months
- not standing with support by 12 months
- not walking by 18 months.

Sometimes, it's simply individual variation but, in some cases, delays may suggest issues with muscle tone, co-ordination, or underlying neurological conditions. Early physiotherapy can make a big difference.

Fine-motor delays

Fine motor skills involve smaller movements, such as grasping objects, feeding with a spoon, or scribbling. Signs to watch for:

- difficulty picking up small objects by 12 months
- not pointing or using fingers to indicate interest by 15 months
- trouble manipulating toys or using utensils by age two.

Fine-motor delays might stem from muscle-tone issues, hand-eye co-ordination problems, or broader developmental conditions.

Speech and language delays

Language development includes both expressive (speaking) and receptive (understanding) skills. Signs to watch for:

- no babbling by 12 months
- not saying single words by 18 months
- no simple two-word phrases by age two
- not responding to their name consistently or seeming not to understand simple commands.

Delays might be linked to hearing issues, developmental-language disorders, or neurodevelopmental conditions, such as autism. Early referral to speech-and-language therapy can be extremely beneficial.

What should you do if you're worried?

If something doesn't feel right, trust your instincts. You know your child best.

- Talk to your GP or public-health nurse: In both Ireland and the UK, your GP or public-health nurse is your first point of contact. They can carry out developmental screenings, listen to your concerns, and make referrals if needed.
- Keep up with health checks: Attend routine developmental checks, such as the 6–8-week check and the 2–2.5-year review. These appointments are designed to spot issues early.
- Don't 'wait and see': It's a common piece of advice, but not always helpful. While many children do 'catch up', early intervention, even if only precautionary, is better than delay. Getting help early does not label a child, it supports them in reaching their potential.

- Ask for referrals: Depending on the concern, your child may benefit from:
  - physiotherapy (for motor delays)
  - occupational therapy (for fine-motor or sensory issues)
  - speech-and-language therapy
  - developmental paediatric assessment.

I know how easy it is to worry about whether your child is 'on track', but milestones are tools, not tests. They help guide us to spot when a child might need extra support. And if that's the case, it is not a reflection on you as a parent, nor is it a sign your child won't thrive. With the right support, most children can and do make wonderful progress. (See Chapter 9 for more on developmental differences.)

ECZEMA

Eczema is a chronic inflammatory skin condition that causes dry, itchy, and, sometimes, weeping or cracked skin. It often begins in infancy or early childhood and can fluctuate in severity over time. (I also spoke about eczema on page 283.)

Signs and symptoms

In babies and young children, eczema typically presents as:

- dry, rough, or scaly patches on the face, scalp, and body
- redness and inflammation, especially in the creases of the elbows, behind the knees, or on the wrists and ankles
- itching (often severe), which can lead to scratching, broken skin, and sleep disturbances
- oozing or crusting skin during flare-ups
- thickened skin (lichenification) over time due to persistent scratching.

In infants under six months, eczema often affects the cheeks and forehead first. In toddlers and older children, it tends to settle into the flexural areas (elbows, knees, neck).

Causes and risk factors

Eczema is not contagious. It's caused by a combination of genetic and environmental factors. Children are more likely to develop the condition if there's a family history of eczema, asthma, or hay fever (the 'atopic triad').

A child with eczema has a compromised skin barrier, meaning the skin doesn't retain moisture well and is more susceptible to irritants, allergens, and infections.

Common triggers

Triggers vary from child to child, but some common ones include the following:

- cold, dry weather, particularly relevant in Irish and UK winters
- soaps and bubble baths, as even those marketed for children can irritate
- wool or synthetic clothing: rough fabrics can worsen itching
- heat and sweating
- dust mites, pet dander, or pollen
- food allergies in some children, particularly under one year old. Cow's milk, eggs, and peanuts are common culprits
- stress and illness: even toddlers can react physically to emotional and physical stress.

Treatment

There is no cure for eczema, but it can be managed effectively. Treatment focuses on maintaining the skin barrier and controlling inflammation.

Daily skincare routine
- Use fragrance-free emollients several times a day (especially after bathing).
- Avoid soaps; use soap substitutes or gentle cleansers.
- Keep baths short (5–10 minutes) and use lukewarm water.

Topical steroids
- For flare-ups, topical corticosteroids are essential (used under medical supervision).
- Use the right strength for the right area (for example, milder for the face).
- When used appropriately, they are safe and effective.

Antihistamines
- These can be useful at night if itching disrupts sleep, though they don't treat the eczema itself.

Treating infections
- Broken skin can become infected with bacteria, such as Staphylococcus aureus.
- Look for signs like yellow crusting, pus, or rapidly worsening redness.
- Your GP may prescribe antibiotic creams or oral antibiotics if needed.

Seek medical advice in each of the following cases:

- **eczema that isn't improving despite good skincare and emollients**
- **signs of infection, such as:**
  - **weeping or yellow crusts**
  - **pus-filled spots**
  - **fever with skin symptoms**
- **sudden worsening of eczema or whole-body redness**
- **eyes are affected, such as swelling, pain, or discharge**
- **concerns about allergy or food triggers, particularly in very young children or those with a history of reactions.**

Managing eczema can feel overwhelming, especially when it's severe or persistent. Don't be afraid to ask questions and always seek a review if your child's eczema isn't responding. Early, effective treatment eases discomfort and helps prevent long-term complications.

EYES

Why have my toddler's eyes turned red?
Does my baby have a squint?
Can my preschooler see properly?
The appearance of your child's eyes can often cause you to ask yourself, 'Is this normal or is there something funny going on with their eyes?'

From the moment your baby opens their eyes, you'll notice their world slowly coming into focus. Vision plays a crucial role in a child's development. That's why it's so important to be aware of normal eye development and the signs that something might not be quite right.

Is it normal for a newborn to squint?

Yes, in the early weeks of life, it's common for newborns to appear slightly cross-eyed or for their eyes not to move in perfect co-ordination. This usually improves as their eye muscles strengthen, typically by around six to eight weeks of age. However, if you continue to notice a squint (one eye turning in, out, up, or down) after three months of age, it's a good idea to seek professional advice.

Persistent squinting can affect vision development and may be a sign of a condition called 'strabismus', which can lead to amblyopia (lazy eye) if untreated.

Can babies be born with cataracts?

Yes, although rare, some babies are born with cataracts (clouding of the eye's lens). These are called 'congenital cataracts', and they can affect one or both eyes. They may be inherited or linked to certain infections or conditions during pregnancy. If cataracts are dense or large, they can significantly impair a baby's vision and need prompt assessment by a paediatric ophthalmologist (eye specialist).

In Ireland and the UK, newborns undergo a routine eye examination as part of the newborn examination to help detect cataracts early.

What does it mean if my baby's pupils don't look red in photos?

You've probably noticed how camera flashes often create a red-eye effect in photos. This red glow is actually a reflection of the retina – and it's a good thing! If one or both eyes show a white, yellow, or unusually dark reflection (called 'leukocoria') instead of red, it could be a sign of a serious eye problem, such as:

- congenital cataracts
- retinoblastoma (a rare childhood eye cancer)
- a retinal abnormality.

If you notice this in a photo, it's worth getting checked promptly by your GP.

What should I do if I think my child has a squint or vision problem?

If you're concerned about your child's eyes – maybe one eye seems to turn, or your child is bumping into things or not making eye contact – trust your instincts. Early intervention is key. Here's what to do:

- Speak to your GP: They can refer you to an orthoptist or paediatric ophthalmologist if needed.
- Children's vision screening: In Ireland and the UK, children are typically screened between the ages of four and five years as part of school-entry checks. However, don't wait for this if you suspect a problem earlier.
- Don't delay: The earlier problems like amblyopia or strabismus are treated, the better the outcome.

Eye infections in babies and children

Children are prone to a number of eye infections, which can range from mild to serious:

- Conjunctivitis (pink eye): This is common and usually caused by viruses or bacteria. Symptoms include red, sticky,

itchy eyes. Most mild cases clear on their own, but bacterial cases may need antibiotic drops.
- Uveitis: Inflammation of the middle layer of the eye. This is less common but more serious and often linked to underlying health conditions, such as juvenile arthritis. It can cause pain, redness, light sensitivity, and blurred vision.
- Periorbital cellulitis: A serious bacterial infection of the tissues around the eye. Signs include swelling, redness, and tenderness around the eyelid. It may follow a sinus or skin infection. This condition needs urgent medical attention.

Contact your GP, out-of-hours service, or attend the ED without delay if you notice any of the following:

- **a white, grey or yellow pupil in photos or in real life**
- **a persistent squint beyond three months of age**
- **one or both eyes not tracking or responding to movement/light**
- **signs of eye pain, extreme light sensitivity, or vision loss**
- **redness and swelling around the eye, especially if it's painful or your child seems unwell**
- **cloudiness in the eye or change in the size/shape of the pupil**
- **unusual eye movements (e.g. eyes flicking side to side constantly).**

Most eye issues in children are treatable, but timing matters. As a parent or caregiver, you're in the best position to spot early signs of any issues, so don't hesitate to speak up if something doesn't seem right.

FEVER

Fever is not an illness in itself, it is a symptom. It is a higher-than-normal body temperature, typically 38°C or above, and is usually a sign of infection.

Most fevers in children are caused by viruses, such as colds, flu, or other seasonal bugs. Sometimes, it's a bacterial infection, such as a UTI or tonsillitis. Occasionally, fever can be a sign of something more serious, like sepsis.

How to measure a temperature accurately

The most accurate method of measuring temperature depends on your child's age:

- Under three months: A fever at this age is always taken seriously. At home, use an underarm digital thermometer. Your baby will have to be checked out in a medical setting, and the doctors or nurses may use a rectal thermometer.
- Three months to five years: A digital thermometer under the armpit works best.
- Over five years: You can use a digital thermometer in the mouth, or a well-positioned ear thermometer.

Avoid forehead strips as they are not reliable. And steer clear of old-style mercury thermometers – they're unsafe!

Personally, I never invested in a fancy, expensive thermometer. I always just used the simple little digital thermometers you can pick up in the pharmacy.

Do I always need to treat a fever?

When it comes to temperatures, keep the saying 'treat the child, not the number' in mind. If your child has a temperature of 38°C but is happy, playing, drinking and alert, you don't need to bring the fever down with medicine. On the other hand, a child with a mild fever who is miserable and off form might need some help.

You can use paracetamol (such as Calpol) or ibuprofen (such as Nurofen) as appropriate for your child's age and weight if your child is:

- uncomfortable or in pain
- not drinking or sleeping
- miserable and unsettled.

What's normal with fever? What's not?

It's completely normal for children with a fever to:

- be flushed and warm
- feel tired or clingy
- eat and drink less
- sleep more.

However, trust your gut if something feels 'off'.

Seek urgent medical help if your child:

- is very drowsy or hard to wake
- has fast or laboured breathing
- has a rash that doesn't fade when pressed

- has a stiff neck or light sensitivity
- has a seizure, especially a first-time febrile seizure
- has cold hands and feet with a hot body
- is under three months and has any fever at all
- is crying persistently or has high-pitched screaming
- has no wet nappies or there are signs of dehydration.

If your child has a fever, but no red flags:

- Keep them hydrated – offer water or milk frequently.
- Dress them in light clothing and keep the room well ventilated.
- Let them rest, but don't worry if they perk up and want to play.
- Keep a close eye on them – especially at night.

You don't need to sponge them down or cool them with fans; it's better to let the body manage its own temperature unless they're very uncomfortable.

When to call the doctor

Call your GP or out-of-hours service if:

- the fever lasts more than five days
- your child is getting worse, not better
- you're worried about how your child is breathing, behaving, or drinking
- your child is not responding to fever-reducing medicine
- your child is under three months and has any fever at all.

Fever can be frightening but, in most cases, it's part of the body's normal defence against infection. A raised temperature alone isn't dangerous, and you don't always need to act on it.

Always focus on how your child is acting: if they are alert, feeding, and comforted by you, that matters more than the reading on the thermometer.

GASTROENTERITIS

Gastroenteritis is an infection of the gut, usually caused by viruses, such as rotavirus or norovirus. Occasionally, it can be due to bacteria, such as Salmonella or E. coli, or parasites, though these are less common in Ireland and the UK.

It spreads easily, especially in childcare settings, and can affect children of all ages. The immune systems of babies and toddlers are still developing, which makes them more vulnerable to the effects of dehydration.

Symptoms

Symptoms typically appear within one to three days of infection and can last for up to a week. They include:

- diarrhoea, often watery and frequent
- vomiting, sometimes sudden and forceful
- fever, mild to moderate
- abdominal pain or cramps
- loss of appetite and general irritability
- lethargy: your child may seem more tired or subdued than usual.

How to manage gastroenteritis at home

In most cases, gastroenteritis can be managed at home with rest and hydration.

- **Fluids first:** Offer small, frequent sips of fluid. Water or oral rehydration solutions, such as Dioralyte, are ideal. Breastfed babies should continue to breastfeed. Formula-fed babies can usually continue their usual feeds. Avoid fizzy drinks or fruit juices, which can worsen diarrhoea.
- **Keep feeding if possible:** There's no need to stop food for most children. Offer bland, easy-to-digest foods like toast, plain pasta, mashed potato, or rice when vomiting settles.
- **Hygiene matters:** Wash hands thoroughly after nappy changes or toilet visits. Disinfect surfaces and wash clothes and bedding promptly.

Young children can become dehydrated quickly, so watch out for the following signs:

- dry mouth or tongue
- sunken eyes or a sunken soft spot (fontanelle) in babies
- less frequent wet nappies or no urine for over six hours
- dark, concentrated urine
- lethargy, drowsiness, or irritability
- cool hands and feet.

While most children recover well, you should seek urgent medical help if your child:

- **has signs of moderate to severe dehydration**
- **is under three months old and has vomiting or diarrhoea**
- **has bloody diarrhoea**
- **is vomiting persistently and unable to keep any fluids down**
- **becomes very drowsy, floppy, or difficult to wake**

- **has a high fever (over 39°C), especially in a baby under six months**
- **has a seizure or fit**
- **shows signs of severe pain or a swollen tummy.**

Gastroenteritis is unpleasant but usually resolves itself. The key is maintaining hydration, monitoring for red flags, and giving your child plenty of rest.

Always trust your instincts – if something doesn't feel right, contact your GP, out-of-hours service, or emergency services.

HAIR

Parents worry about hair. Does my baby have too much hair? Too little? Why is their hair falling out? Is this normal? Let me reassure you, in most cases, it absolutely is normal.

Hair growth in children is incredibly varied, and what's 'normal' spans a wide range. But there are times when slower growth, sudden thinning, or bald patches may need a second look.

Hair development begins in the womb, at around 14 weeks' gestation. However, whether your baby is born with a luscious mane or just a soft fuzz is largely down to genetics. Even if your baby is born with a full head of hair, don't be surprised if they lose it within the first few months. This is entirely normal and brings us to a phenomenon called 'telogen effluvium'.

What is telogen effluvium?

Telogen effluvium is a common, temporary hair loss that happens when a major stress (such as birth) pushes a large number of hair follicles into the 'resting' phase. After a few months, those hairs fall out all at once.

In babies, this often occurs at around 8–12 weeks of age and may result in bald patches (especially at the back of the head, due to friction against mattresses). New hair usually grows back over the coming months, though it might be a different colour or texture.

What if my toddler's hair still isn't growing?

While some toddlers have thick, fast-growing hair early on, others remain fine-haired or sparse-headed until preschool age. Again, much of this is genetic.

However, a lack of hair growth beyond age two or three, especially if accompanied by other symptoms like poor growth, dry skin, or developmental delay, may warrant further evaluation. Nutritional deficiencies (particularly iron, zinc, or biotin), thyroid issues, or genetic conditions can occasionally impact hair growth.

If your child's hair seems unusually sparse or not growing at all by age three, it's worth discussing it with your GP or paediatrician.

Why does hair sometimes fall out or thin suddenly?

Sudden thinning in toddlers or preschoolers is most often still linked to telogen effluvium, which can be triggered by high fevers, surgery, infections, or emotional stress – even weeks after the event. Again, it's temporary, and hair regrowth typically resumes within three to six months.

What about bald patches?

If you notice round or oval bald patches, especially with smooth, non-scaly skin, this could be a sign of alopecia areata. This is an autoimmune condition where the immune system attacks the hair follicles. It's not painful, and children are otherwise healthy.

Alopecia areata affects about 1–2% of people and often starts in childhood. It may resolve on its own or persist. While there is no cure, treatments are available to encourage regrowth, and support from dermatology specialists is important.

Another common cause of patchy hair loss is scalp ringworm, a fungal infection (see page 288 for more details). This often shows as a scaly patch of hair loss and may be itchy. It spreads easily in preschools and crèches. If you suspect this, your child will need an antifungal medicine. Topical creams are not enough.

Why do some children pull out their hair?

Trichotillomania is a compulsive habit of pulling out your own hair, sometimes without realising it. It's more common in children over three and can be a response to stress, anxiety, or even boredom.

Hair loss in these cases often appears uneven or with broken hairs of different lengths. Trichotillomania can be short-lived, or it can persist and require psychological support or behavioural therapy.

What about body hair?

Is it normal for babies and toddlers to have hair on their back, arms and legs? Yes, in most cases, it's perfectly normal.

Many newborns are born with lanugo, a fine, downy hair that covers the back, shoulders, and, sometimes, even the forehead or ears. This is more common in premature babies and usually disappears within the first few weeks of life.

As children grow, body hair on the arms, legs, and back can vary greatly depending on ethnicity and genetics. Some children naturally have more visible or darker hair than others, and that's not a cause for concern.

When it comes to underarm or pubic hair, however, it is different. Hair growth in areas such as the underarms or pubic region before the age of eight in girls and nine in boys is not typical, and it could be a sign of precocious (abnormally early) puberty, where the body starts maturing earlier than expected.

It's not always serious, but it does need to be assessed. Early signs of puberty should be evaluated by a doctor to rule out underlying hormonal imbalances or conditions affecting the adrenal or pituitary glands. So, if you notice the following, make an appointment with your GP or paediatrician:

- pubic or underarm hair before age eight (girls) and nine (boys)
- breast development or testicular enlargement
- rapid growth in height
- body odour or acne in very young children.

In most cases, it's manageable and treatable, and early evaluation helps.

When to seek medical advice

You should speak to your GP or paediatrician if:

- your child's hair isn't growing by age two to three
- there are sudden bald patches, especially if they're smooth or circular
- you notice scaling, redness, or itching on the scalp
- hair is falling out in clumps
- your child pulls out their own hair or eyelashes
- there are early signs of puberty
- there are other symptoms, such as fatigue, poor appetite, or skin changes.

Hair patterns in children vary widely, but if you have a concern or a question about your child's hair – either on their head or on their body – don't hesitate to ask.

HAYFEVER

Springtime brings longer days, flowers in bloom, and – for many children – the dreaded sniffles, itchy eyes, and sneezes that seem never-ending. Hayfever, also called allergic rhinitis, affects many children. Understanding it can help you spot it early, manage symptoms effectively, and even consider long-term treatments.

What causes hayfever?

Hayfever is caused by the immune system overreacting to harmless substances in the environment, usually pollen from trees, grasses, or weeds. When a child's body encounters pollen, it treats it as a threat and releases chemicals such as histamine, causing the familiar hayfever symptoms.

Environmental triggers can include:

- tree pollen (common in spring)
- grass pollen (common in late spring and early summer)
- weed pollen (more common in late summer).

Symptoms can range from mild to severe, and often include:

- sneezing and runny or blocked nose
- itchy, watery eyes
- cough or sore throat from post-nasal drip
- fatigue or irritability due to disrupted sleep.

Unlike a cold, hayfever is seasonal (though some children may have symptoms year-round) and usually doesn't cause a fever.

How is hayfever diagnosed?

Diagnosis typically starts with your GP or a paediatrician asking about your child's symptoms and when they occur. They may also recommend:

- Skin-prick tests: Small amounts of allergens are placed on the skin to see if a reaction occurs.
- Blood tests: Measures levels of specific antibodies (IgE) linked to allergies.

Accurate diagnosis helps pinpoint the trigger and guides treatment.

Managing hayfever

Most children find relief with a combination of strategies:
Avoidance:

- Keep windows closed on high pollen days.
- Shower and change clothes after playing outdoors.
- Don't dry clothes outdoors during peak pollen season.
- Wear a hat and wraparound sunglasses when outside to reduce pollen contact.
- Wash hair before bed to remove pollen.

Medications:

- Oral antihistamines (relieve sneezing, itching, and runny nose)
- Nasal steroid sprays (reduce inflammation and congestion)
- Eye drops for itchy or watery eyes

Long-term treatments: Immunotherapy

For children with moderate to severe hayfever, allergen immunotherapy (sometimes called 'desensitisation' or 'allergy shots') may offer long-term relief. This is a specialised treatment that is usually prescribed by a paediatric allergist.

- Usually recommended for: Children aged five and above, though age limits may vary depending on the type of therapy.
- How it works: Small, gradually increasing doses of the allergen are given over time (either as injections or under-the-tongue tablets). This helps the immune system become less sensitive to the allergen, potentially reducing symptoms for years.
- Duration: Typically lasts three–five years for full effect.

Immunotherapy is especially helpful if your child's symptoms are not controlled by medications or significantly affect daily life, school, or sleep.

While hayfever can be frustrating, early recognition and a combination of avoidance, medication, and possibly immunotherapy, when your child is older, can make a big difference. Keeping a diary of your child's symptoms, noting triggers, and talking to your GP or a paediatric allergy specialist can help your family enjoy the spring and summer months more comfortably.

HEAD LICE

I guarantee you that your scalp will feel itchy after reading this section, so apologies in advance!

Head lice (or Pediculus humanus capitis) are small, wingless insects that live in the hair and feed on blood from the scalp. They're about the size of a sesame seed, and their eggs, called 'nits', are even smaller, appearing as tiny white or yellowish dots attached firmly to the hair shaft, often near the scalp.

Contrary to some myths, head lice do not jump or fly. They crawl, and they survive by close contact.

How do they spread?

In toddlers and young children, lice usually spread through head-to-head contact, which is common during play, cuddles, or naps. Sharing hats, brushes, or bedding can also spread lice, but this is a much less common way for them to spread.

Head lice are not a sign of poor hygiene. They don't care whether hair is clean or dirty, long or short.

How to spot head lice

In many cases, the first sign is itching, although not everyone gets this straightaway. Other signs include:

- seeing live lice in the hair or crawling on the scalp
- finding nits (eggs), especially behind the ears and at the nape of the neck
- irritability or trouble sleeping – lice are more active at night
- red bite marks or sores from scratching.

For toddlers, who may not be able to express what they're feeling, you might just notice extra scratching or discomfort.

How are head lice treated?

There are two main approaches to treatment: medicated treatments and manual removal.

Medicated treatments

These are available from your local pharmacy in the form of lotions, sprays, or shampoos. In Ireland and the UK, common over-the-counter treatments include dimeticone-based products that work by physically coating and suffocating the lice.

- Always follow the instructions carefully.

- A second application is usually recommended seven days after the first to catch any newly hatched lice.
- Not all treatments are suitable for young children. Check the age guidelines or ask your pharmacist or GP for advice if your child is under two.

Wet combing

This is a chemical-free method involving:

- washing the hair with conditioner
- combing through hair with a fine-toothed lice comb, section by section
- repeating every three to four days for at least two weeks.

This method requires persistence but it can be effective if you prefer to avoid medicated treatment.

Does my child need to see a doctor?

Most cases of head lice do not need a visit to the GP. However, you should seek medical advice if:

- you're unsure if what you're seeing is lice
- over-the-counter treatments aren't working
- your child has signs of infection (redness or swelling on the scalp, pus-filled spots or sores, fever, or is generally feeling unwell)
- your child has eczema or other skin conditions that make treatment more difficult.

In rare cases, intense scratching can break the skin and lead to secondary bacterial infections, such as impetigo, which may require antibiotics.

Can we prevent head lice?

Unfortunately, there's no guaranteed way to prevent head lice. However, some helpful tips include:

- regular checks, especially if you know there's an outbreak at your child's school or crèche
- keeping long hair tied back
- avoiding sharing hairbrushes, hats, or pillows.

There's limited evidence that repellent sprays or tea tree oils work, and they can sometimes irritate young skin, so, if you use these, do so with caution.

It's easy to feel overwhelmed or even embarrassed when you find head lice on your child, but you are not alone, and there's nothing to be ashamed of. Head lice are a normal part of childhood in communal settings and not a reflection of parenting or hygiene.

MEASLES

Measles is a highly contagious viral infection caused by the measles virus. It primarily affects children, but it can strike at any age if a person isn't immune. It begins with cold-like symptoms but quickly escalates, making it far more serious than a simple childhood illness.

Symptoms

Symptoms usually appear about 10 days after exposure and may include:

- high fever (over 38°C)
- cough, runny nose, and red, watery eyes (conjunctivitis)

- Koplik spots (tiny white spots inside the mouth)
- a rash, starting on the face and behind the ears, spreading down the body.

Children are often extremely unwell during this time, with fatigue, loss of appetite, and irritability.

How does it spread?

Measles spreads through airborne droplets when someone with the virus coughs or sneezes. The virus can survive on surfaces for up to two hours. It's so infectious that up to 9 in 10 unvaccinated people who come into contact with someone infected will catch it.

Hospitalisation and complications

Measles is not just a rash and a fever. It can lead to serious complications, especially in children under five, pregnant women, and those with weakened immune systems.

- Around one in five children with measles will require hospitalisation.
- Common complications include ear infections, pneumonia, and diarrhoea.
- More severe risks include:
  - encephalitis (brain inflammation) – this can cause seizures, brain damage, or death
  - blindness or permanent hearing loss
  - subacute sclerosing panencephalitis (SSPE) – a rare but fatal brain disorder that can develop years after measles infection.

Why is measles on the rise?

There are several factors behind the resurgence in measles:

- Falling vaccine uptake: In some areas, MMR (measles, mumps, rubella) coverage has dropped below 85%, well short of the 95% target needed for herd immunity.
- Misinformation about vaccines, especially online, continues to sow doubt about their safety.
- COVID-19 disruptions led to missed or delayed routine vaccinations.
- Increased international travel also contributes to the spread.

MMR vaccine guidelines

In both Ireland and the UK, the MMR vaccine is part of the routine childhood immunisation schedule:

- First dose: At 12–13 months of age.
- Second dose: Usually in the first year of primary school, aged 4–5.

These two doses provide about 99% protection against measles. For children born on or after 1 October 2024 in Ireland, the booster vaccine in primary school will be called the MMRV, and it will include the varicella (chickenpox) vaccine.

What if your child is under one?

Infants under one year are too young for routine MMR, but in certain high-risk situations, such as travel to outbreak areas or known exposure, they can receive the vaccine as early as six months.

However, this early dose doesn't count towards the two scheduled doses. This is because maternal antibodies (passed from mum during pregnancy) may interfere with the vaccine's effectiveness in very young babies. That's why two further doses are still needed at the usual ages to ensure lasting immunity.

What can parents do?

To protect your child against contracting measles do the following:

- Check your child's vaccination status with your GP.
- Catch up on any missed doses – it's never too late to get vaccinated.
- For babies under one who may be travelling abroad or have been exposed to measles, ask your doctor about early vaccination.
- Stay vigilant for symptoms and keep unwell children home to prevent spread.

Measles is not just a childhood nuisance, it's a serious illness with potentially devastating consequences. Fortunately, it's also preventable. Vaccination remains your best defence, not only protecting your child but helping to shield vulnerable members of the community.

NAPPY RASH AND THRUSH

Nappy rash (also called diaper dermatitis) is inflammation of the skin in the nappy area. It is very common, affecting up to a third of nappy-wearing babies at any one time. (I also spoke about nappy rash on page 88.)

Nappy rash is caused by:

- prolonged exposure to wetness (urine or stools)
- friction from nappies
- sensitivity to products, such as baby wipes, soaps, or detergents

- illness or teething, which can make stools more acidic
- antibiotic use, which can disrupt the skin's natural barrier.

Symptoms

If your child has nappy rash, they might show the following signs:

- Red or pink patches on the skin, usually on the buttocks, thighs, and genitals.
- The skin may look sore, shiny, or slightly raised.
- It can vary from a few small spots to large areas of irritated skin.
- Your baby may be fussier than usual, especially during nappy changes.

How is it treated?

To treat nappy rash, you can do the following:

- Frequent nappy changes – keep the area as dry as possible.
- Gentle cleaning – use warm water and cotton wool or fragrance-free wipes.
- Air time – let your baby go nappy-free for short periods.
- Barrier creams – zinc-based creams, such as Sudocrem, Bepanthen, or Metanium, protect and soothe the skin.
- Avoid irritants – don't use perfumed wipes, bubble baths, or harsh soaps.

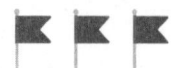

See your GP or public-health nurse if:

- the rash doesn't improve after three to five days of home treatment

What about thrush?

Thrush (caused by a yeast, Candida albicans) often develops on top of a nappy rash, especially after antibiotic use or if the rash has been lingering for more than a few days.

It is caused by:

- a moist, warm environment under the nappy that enables yeast to thrive
- antibiotics (taken by either a baby or a breastfeeding mum) that can kill beneficial bacteria, letting yeast overgrow.

Symptoms

The following can be signs of thrush:

- bright red rash with defined edges
- small satellite spots just outside the main rash area
- skin is often shiny, inflamed, and may look raw
- doesn't typically respond to barrier creams alone.

How is thrush treated?

You can use the following to treat thrush:

Antifungal cream, such as clotrimazole or miconazole, prescribed by your GP or pharmacist. Apply twice daily for at least 7–10 days, even if the rash improves.

- the skin becomes broken, weepy, or oozes pus
- there are blisters or ulcers
- your baby develops a fever
- the rash appears suddenly and spreads quickly.

Tips to prevent nappy rash and thrush

To prevent your child developing nappy rash and thrush, you can do the following:

- Change nappies promptly, especially after poos.
- Let your baby's skin air dry when possible.
- Use barrier creams regularly if your baby is prone to rashes.
- Choose breathable nappies and avoid tight clothing.
- Wash cloth nappies thoroughly and rinse well.
- Treat oral thrush in your baby (or yourself if you are breastfeeding) to prevent reinfection.

Most nappy rashes are mild and respond well to simple changes. However, if you're concerned that the rash looks angry, is not healing, or is causing your baby distress, don't hesitate to seek advice. Infections, particularly fungal ones like thrush, need specific treatment and won't get better on their own.

Feature	Nappy Rash	Thrush
Appearance	Red, sore, flat, or slightly raised areas	Red, shiny rash with distinct edges
Spots beyond rash	Usually absent	Yes – 'satellite' spots or pimples
Response to barrier cream	Often improves within days	Doesn't improve or worsens
Cause	Irritation, wetness	Yeast, often after antibiotics or prolonged rash
Treatment	Barrier cream, air time	Antifungal cream required

In severe cases, an oral antifungal may be needed.

POISONING AND ACCIDENTAL INGESTION

I know how frightening it can be to suspect that your child might have swallowed something dangerous. To prevent this as much as possible, ensure you store all dangerous items securely and out of reach of your child.

Common household hazards for under fives

Keep these locked away and out of sight:

- medicines and vitamins
- cleaning products and laundry/dishwasher pods
- garden chemicals and fertilisers
- cosmetics, perfumes, and deodorants
- batteries (especially button cells)
- essential oils and air fresheners
- alcohol (even small amounts)
- cigarettes and e-cigarettes
- firelighters
- toxic plants and wild mushrooms
- needles and syringes.

Avoid calling medicine 'sweets' as this can confuse your child – children copy what they see and hear.
Here's what to do if your child does ingest something dangerous:

Act promptly – don't wait

In Ireland, call the National Poisons Information Centre (NPIC) at 01 809 2166 (available 8am – 10pm). Their trained staff will assess the situation and advise whether urgent medical attention is needed. They may refer you to the nearest emergency department. If it's outside these hours, call your GP or go straight to the nearest emergency department.

Have the following information ready when you call the helpline or arrive at the hospital:

- what your child ingested or injected – keep the container or label
- approximate amount they took
- the time it happened
- your child's age, weight, and current symptoms.

Never induce vomiting

It's natural to think you should 'get it out', but vomiting can make things worse, especially if the substance is corrosive or if it could be inhaled into the lungs. Wait for professional advice.

Button batteries are a true emergency

If you suspect your child has swallowed a button battery, go straight to the emergency department – tissue damage can begin within minutes.

For children over one year old, and only if they can swallow safely, you may give two teaspoons of honey while on the way to the ED. This coats the battery and may slow damage – but don't delay hospital care.

After the incident

After your child has received the help they need:

- Watch for any delayed symptoms.
- Follow up with your GP if advised.
- Reassess home safety to prevent future accidents.

SEPSIS

'Sepsis' is one of those medical terms that can sound terrifying. It's a condition that moves fast and can have serious consequences, especially for children under five. But the good news is that when caught early, sepsis is treatable. The key is awareness.

So, let's talk about what it is, what signs to watch for, and what to do if you feel your concerns aren't being taken seriously.

What is sepsis?

Sepsis is the body's extreme response to an infection. Rather than fighting off germs in a controlled way, the immune system goes into overdrive and starts attacking its own tissues and organs. In small children, whose immune systems are still developing, this can escalate rapidly.

Sepsis is not caused by one specific bug. It can be triggered by common infections such as urinary tract infections, skin infections, or even a bad case of flu or chickenpox. It's not the infection itself that's the problem, it's how the body responds to it.

Who is most at risk?

Children under five are among the most vulnerable. Their immune systems are still learning how to handle infections. Babies under one year, children with weakened immune systems, and those with recent surgery or medical devices, such as central lines or catheters, are at particular risk.

Signs and symptoms of sepsis

The symptoms of sepsis can mimic those of many common illnesses, but trust your instincts – if something feels 'off', seek help. Warning signs include:

- breathing very fast
- having a fit or convulsion
- looking mottled, bluish, or pale
- being very lethargic or difficult to wake
- feeling abnormally cold to the touch
- not feeding or showing no interest in feeding
- vomiting repeatedly or not keeping feeds down
- not passing urine or having fewer wet nappies than usual
- a rash that doesn't fade when pressed with a clear glass.

Remember, not all symptoms have to be present. Even one or two of these signs is enough to raise concern.

How urgent is it?

Very. Sepsis is a medical emergency. Early treatment makes all the difference. If caught early, children usually recover well with antibiotics and fluids. But if left too long, it can lead to organ failure, limb loss, or even death.

If you suspect sepsis, don't wait. Go to the emergency department or call 999/112. Tell the medical team, 'I'm worried this could be sepsis.' It helps prioritise care.

How is sepsis treated?

Treatment for sepsis typically starts with:

- immediate antibiotics, given through a drip (IV)
- intravenous fluids to support blood pressure and hydration

oxygen if your child is struggling to breathe
• close monitoring in hospital, often in a high-dependency or intensive-care unit in severe cases.

The earlier treatment begins, the better the outcome. Most children recover fully, but speed is crucial.

What if your concerns are not being heard?

This is something I feel very strongly about as a paediatrician and as a parent. You know your child best. If you feel that something is seriously wrong and you're not being taken seriously, do the following:

- Be clear and assertive. Say, 'I'm worried this could be sepsis.'
- Ask for a second opinion. You are entitled to it.
- Ask for observations to be repeated. Vital signs like heart rate, temperature, breathing rate, and oxygen levels can change quickly in young children.
- If in doubt, go back. Don't be afraid to return to the emergency department or call 999/112 if your child gets worse.

In both Ireland and the UK, there are national guidelines in place to help doctors and nurses recognise and treat sepsis. But no system is perfect, and your voice is essential.

Sepsis in children is rare but, when it happens, time is everything. The most important message I want to give you is this: if your child is unwell and seems 'just not right', trust your gut. You are never wasting anyone's time by seeking medical attention.

SUDDEN INFANT DEATH SYNDROME

> **Trigger warning:** This section discusses sudden infant death and may be distressing for some parents or caregivers.

Sudden infant death syndrome (SIDS), sometimes known as 'cot death', is one of the most devastating and deeply feared experiences a parent can face. But with knowledge and support, we can ease some of that anxiety and focus on what matters most: keeping babies as safe as possible, while nurturing their sleep and development.

Let's take a look at how to navigate the balance between vigilance and peace of mind.

What is SIDS?

SIDS refers to the sudden and unexplained death of a seemingly healthy baby, usually during sleep, and typically under the age of one year. It often occurs in infants between two and four months old, and it remains unexplained even after thorough investigation, including postmortem, examination of the death scene, and medical history.

It's important to emphasise that SIDS is rare, but its impact is profound.

Are some babies more at risk?

Yes, while SIDS can occur in any infant, some babies have a higher risk. Risk factors include:

- premature birth or low birth weight
- exposure to smoke during pregnancy or after birth

- gender: boys are slightly more affected than girls
- overheating or head-covering during sleep
- soft bedding or co-sleeping in unsafe conditions
- sleep position: tummy sleeping increases risk.

Importantly, socioeconomic factors, including access to prenatal care and safe sleep education, also play a role.

What does the latest research show?

SIDS remains complex and multifactorial. However, new research offers some hope in better understanding potential causes:

- Brainstem abnormalities: Studies have shown that some babies who die from SIDS may have underlying differences in the areas of the brain that control breathing, arousal, and heart-rate regulation.
- Triple-Risk Model: This widely accepted theory suggests SIDS occurs when three elements overlap:
  - a vulnerable baby (e.g. immature brain development)
  - a critical developmental period
  - external stressors (e.g. illness or tummy sleeping).

Despite years of study, SIDS is not something parents can fully predict or control. This is important to acknowledge, especially for those burdened by guilt or confusion.

Why is safe sleep important?

Safe-sleep guidelines are one of the most effective tools we have to reduce the risk of SIDS. Key recommendations include:

- placing babies on their backs for every sleep
- using a firm, flat sleep surface (cot or Moses basket) with no loose bedding, pillows, or toys

SHOULD I BE WORRIED?

- room-sharing (but not bed-sharing) for the first six months
- keeping the baby's head uncovered and avoiding overheating
- avoiding smoking in pregnancy and around the baby.

These guidelines have led to a dramatic drop in SIDS cases in Ireland and the UK since the early 1990s.

Can SIDS still happen when parents do everything 'right'?

Tragically, yes. In a small number of cases, SIDS can occur even when parents follow every guideline. This is one of the hardest truths to accept.

If you or someone you know has experienced a loss like this, please understand: it is *not your fault*. You did not fail. Sometimes, despite our best efforts, we are left without answers. Remember that support is available and that you are not alone.

What about monitors and devices?

Devices, such as wearable sensor-based monitors, claim to track heart rate and oxygen levels. While they may bring peace of mind to some parents, they are not medical devices and are *not* proven to prevent SIDS.

These devices can sometimes lead to a false sense of security or increased anxiety due to false alarms.

If you choose to use a device, do so with full understanding: it may help ease anxiety, but it is *not* a guarantee.

What if I feel overwhelmed by anxiety about SIDS?

Many parents, especially new parents, feel intense anxiety around sleep and SIDS. That anxiety is valid, but it should not overshadow the joy of bonding with your baby.

Here are some practical steps that might help:

- Stick to a simple, safe sleep routine. Sometimes, structure itself is reassuring.
- Limit internet searching, which can lead to increased anxiety rather than reassurance.
- Talk to your GP or public-health nurse if you're struggling to sleep or constantly feeling afraid.
- Join a parenting group. Hearing others voice similar concerns can be a lifeline.
- Try mindfulness or CBT-based apps designed for new parents.

For some, the fear can become intrusive and may need professional support from perinatal mental-health services. Asking for help is a strength, not a weakness.

SIDS is a deeply emotional topic, but knowledge is power. By understanding the risk factors and following safe-sleep guidelines, you are doing everything you can to protect your baby from SIDS.

TONSILLITIS

Tonsillitis can be caused by viruses or bacteria, with viral infections being far more common, especially in younger children. These are often the same viruses that cause colds or flu. Occasionally, tonsillitis is caused by bacterial infections, the most notable being group A Streptococcus (commonly called 'strep throat'). While it's more common in older children, it can still occur in preschoolers. See also page 183.

There are a few reasons why children under five are particularly prone to tonsillitis:

- Immature immune systems: Young children are still building their immunity, making them more vulnerable to infections.

- Close contact with other children: Germs spread quickly in crèches, preschools, or playgroups.
- Frequent upper respiratory infections: The more colds a child gets, the more likely they are to develop tonsillitis as a secondary infection.

How is tonsillitis treated?

Treatment depends on what's causing the infection.

Viral tonsillitis

- Usually resolves on its own within three to five days.
- Treatment is supportive, focusing on:
  - fluids
  - rest
  - paracetamol or ibuprofen for fever and pain.

Bacterial tonsillitis (especially strep throat)

- May require antibiotics, usually penicillin or amoxicillin.
- If antibiotics prescribed, it's important your child completes the full course, even if they're feeling better.

Most children recover well, with or without antibiotics, but symptoms can make eating and drinking uncomfortable, so hydration is key.

When is a tonsillectomy considered?

Tonsillectomy (surgical removal of the tonsils) is not a first-line treatment and is reserved for specific cases. In Ireland and the UK, the National Institute for Health and Care Excellence (NICE) guidelines help determine when surgery might be appropriate. Surgery may be considered if your child has:

- seven or more episodes of tonsillitis in one year
- five or more episodes per year for two consecutive years

A TO Z | 365

- recurrent infections causing sleep apnoea, loud snoring, or difficulty breathing at night
- difficulty swallowing because of enlarged tonsils.

Surgery is always a decision made jointly between parents, paediatricians, and ENT (ear, nose, and throat) specialists.

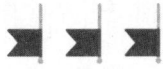

While most cases of tonsillitis are mild, if your child has any of the following signs, they need urgent medical review.

- difficulty breathing or noisy breathing (especially at rest)
- inability to swallow fluids or signs of dehydration (dry lips, no tears when crying, fewer wet nappies)
- high fever that doesn't respond to paracetamol or ibuprofen
- neck stiffness, extreme fatigue, or a child who is hard to wake
- severe throat pain on one side or a swelling of the neck. This could be a sign of a peritonsillar abscess, which is a medical emergency
- if your child appears to be getting worse after a few days, rather than improving.

Tonsillitis can be tough for little ones but, with careful monitoring, pain relief, hydration and antibiotics if needed, most children bounce back quickly.

UNDESCENDED TESTICLES

Undescended testicles (medically known as 'cryptorchidism') is a relatively common condition in baby boys. For parents, it can be worrying to discover that one or both of their baby's testicles are not in the scrotum at birth. However, understanding what's normal, when to be concerned, and what treatment options are available can help you take timely action.

At birth, it's not unusual for one testicle (or both) to not be in the scrotum, particularly in premature babies. Testicular descent typically occurs during the final months of pregnancy, so boys born early are more likely to be born with undescended testicles. Even in full-term babies, about 1 in 30 boys may have at least one undescended testicle at birth. However, in most of these cases, the testicle will descend on its own within the first three to six months of life. Your GP or public-health nurse will check for undescended testicles at your scheduled developmental check-ups.

When should parents be concerned?

If your child's testicle has not descended by six months of age, it's unlikely to do so naturally after that point. In Ireland and the UK, medical guidelines recommend that boys with undescended testicles should be assessed and treated before they are 18 months old.

Parents should also be aware of a condition known as 'retractile testicle', where the testicle moves up and down due to a normal reflex in boys (the cremasteric reflex). This is not the same as an undescended testicle and often resolves without intervention, but it should still be evaluated by a GP or paediatrician to ensure an accurate diagnosis.

When should my child see a specialist?

If a testicle is still not in the scrotum by six months, your GP may refer your child to a paediatric urologist or paediatric surgeon. In Ireland and the UK, HSE and NHS guidelines recommend surgical correction (orchidopexy) to be done ideally before 18 months of age. Early intervention can significantly reduce the risk of complications.

What are the risks of an untreated undescended testicle?

Undescended testicles should not be ignored, as they can lead to several long-term complications:

- Infertility: Testicles that remain in the abdomen or groin are exposed to higher temperatures, which can damage sperm production.
- Increased cancer risk: Men with a history of undescended testicles have a higher risk of testicular cancer, especially if untreated.
- Hernia and testicular torsion: An undescended testicle may be associated with an inguinal hernia or risk of twisting, which is a surgical emergency.
- Psychological impact: As boys get older, having a visible difference in the scrotum can affect self-esteem and body image.

How is it treated?

The main treatment is a surgical procedure called orchidopexy, where the testicle is brought down into the scrotum and fixed in place. This is usually a day-case surgery under general anaesthetic and has a high success rate.

- Surgery is ideally done between 6 and 18 months.
- In some rare cases where the testicle is not found (non-palpable), further imaging or diagnostic laparoscopy may be required.
- If the testicle is missing or underdeveloped, a prosthetic testicle may be considered later in life for cosmetic reasons.

VACCINES

Why are vaccines needed?

Babies are born with immature immune systems. While they receive some antibodies from their mother during pregnancy and breastfeeding, this protection is temporary. Vaccines are designed to teach your baby's immune system how to recognise and fight specific diseases before they ever come into contact with them.

We vaccinate babies early because the diseases we're protecting them from, such as meningitis, whooping cough, measles, and polio, can be especially severe or even fatal in young children.

Vaccination is not just about individual protection, it's about community protection, too. When most people are vaccinated, diseases find it harder to spread. This is called 'herd immunity', and it helps protect those who can't be vaccinated for medical reasons.

Vaccine schedule

I have covered the vaccines administered at each age in the relevant chapters in Part I (see pages 73, 95, 141 and 191), but I have listed the whole current vaccine schedule in Ireland here, including school-age vaccines, to give you the full picture.

For babies born on or after 1 October 2024

At two months
- 6-in-1 (diphtheria, polio, tetanus, pertussis, Hib, hepatitis B)
- PCV
- MenB
- Rotavirus.

At four months
- 6-in-1
- MenB
- Rotavirus.

At six months
- 6-in-1
- PCV.

(MenC is no longer given at this age.)

At 12 months
- MMR
- Chickenpox (varicella)
- MenB.

At 13 months
- 6-in-1
- MenC
- PCV.

Junior infants (four to five years)
- 4-in-1 booster (diphtheria, polio, tetanus, pertussis)
- MMRV (combined MMR and varicella (chickenpox) vaccine).

SHOULD I BE WORRIED?

For children born before 1 October 2024

The vaccines they will receive when they reach school age are as follows:

Junior infants (four to five years)
- 4-in-1 booster (diphtheria, polio, tetanus, pertussis)
- MMR second dose.

First year of secondary school (12 to 14 years)
- HPV
- Tdap booster (tetanus, diphtheria, pertussis)
- MenACWY (meningococcal A, C, W, Y).

Are there risks associated with vaccines?

Like any medical intervention, vaccines can have side-effects. The vast majority are mild and temporary, such as:

- a sore arm
- fever
- fussiness
- mild rash.

Serious side-effects are extremely rare. The risk of a severe allergic reaction (anaphylaxis), for example, is about 1 in 1 million doses. Vaccines are rigorously tested in clinical trials and monitored continually for safety. They must meet incredibly high standards before being approved.

What are the risks of not vaccinating?

Choosing not to vaccinate your child puts them at risk of contracting potentially life-threatening illnesses. Measles, for instance, is highly contagious and can cause complications such as pneumonia, brain inflammation, and even death. In Ireland and the UK, we've seen outbreaks in recent years because vaccination rates have fallen.

It's important to remember that diseases we don't see every day have not disappeared; they are kept at bay by high levels of vaccination.

When the vaccination uptake drops, the diseases will come back.

Why is there so much fear about vaccines?

Social media and the internet are powerful tools for sharing information, but they can also spread misinformation. Unfortunately, many of the most widely circulated vaccine myths are based on outdated, disproven, or deliberately misleading claims. For example, the long-debunked myth linking the MMR vaccine to autism originated from a study that was retracted because of ethical and scientific misconduct. Despite being disproven by countless large-scale studies, the myth still circulates today.

We are wired as humans to protect our children, and that makes us vulnerable to emotionally charged misinformation. The best defence is to seek advice from trusted, qualified professionals and peer-reviewed sources.

Are there dangerous ingredients in vaccines?

No. The ingredients in vaccines are present in tiny, regulated amounts that are safe for babies. Let's clear up a few common concerns:

- Aluminium: Used in some vaccines as an 'adjuvant' to boost the immune response. Babies get more aluminium from breast milk or formula over time than they do from vaccines.
- Formaldehyde: Used in the manufacturing process to inactivate viruses. The trace amounts left in the final vaccine are far less than what naturally occurs in our own bodies.
- Thiomersal (a mercury compound): This is no longer used in routine childhood vaccines in Ireland and the UK. Even when it was, it was used in such tiny amounts that it posed no risk.

Vaccines are among the most scrutinised medical products in the world. Every ingredient is tested for safety, and formulations are constantly reviewed.

If you have concerns about vaccinating your baby, remember the following:

- Vaccines save lives. They are one of the safest and most effective tools in modern medicine.
- The risks of side-effects from vaccines are minimal, especially when compared with the risks of the diseases they prevent.
- Misinformation online is dangerous. Always get your health advice from reputable sources.
- Speak to your GP, public-health nurse, or paediatrician about your concerns. We're here to listen, not judge.

VAGINAL DISCHARGE

Vaginal discharge in baby girls and toddlers can be an unexpected discovery for parents. However, it's not always a cause for concern. Understanding what's normal, what might require medical attention, and how to manage it can help reassure parents and ensure their little ones receive the right care.

'Vaginal discharge' refers to any fluid that comes from a girl's vagina. In babies and toddlers, this can range from clear or white secretions to a small amount of yellowish or slightly blood-tinged fluid. While it may seem unusual, it is often completely normal, especially in infants.

What causes it?

There are several reasons a girl might experience vaginal discharge, many of which are harmless.

Maternal hormones

- Newborn girls may have vaginal discharge or even light vaginal bleeding (often called 'pseudomenstruation') within the first few weeks after birth. This is due to the mother's hormones that pass through the placenta during pregnancy and stimulate the baby's reproductive system.
- This type of discharge usually disappears within a few weeks.

Normal development

- As girls grow, the vaginal area begins producing small amounts of discharge. In toddlers, this can occasionally be seen in the nappy or on underwear.
- A small amount of clear or white discharge without other symptoms is typically normal.

A TO Z | 373

Irritation or hygiene issues

- Poor wiping technique (especially wiping back to front), bubble baths, soaps, or tight clothing can irritate the vaginal area and lead to discharge.
- Nappies and wipes with perfumes can also cause inflammation, known as vulvovaginitis, which may present with discharge.

Infections

- Occasionally, bacterial or yeast infections can cause abnormal discharge. This may be accompanied by redness, soreness, itching, or a strong odour.
- Threadworms, which are common in young children, can also cause irritation and discharge (see page 376 for more details on worms).

Foreign bodies

- Very rarely, toddlers may insert small objects (such as bits of toilet paper) into their vagina, which can cause discharge, often foul-smelling or tinged with blood.

When to see a doctor

Most cases of vaginal discharge in babies and toddlers are mild and harmless. However, medical advice should be sought if:

- the discharge is foul-smelling or green/yellow
- there is persistent redness, swelling, or itching
- your child is unusually fussy or in pain, especially when peeing
- there is bleeding outside the first few weeks of life
- there is any sign of a foreign object or trauma
- the discharge lasts more than a few days or keeps returning.

Your GP or paediatrician may perform a gentle physical examination and may take a swab if infection is suspected.

How is it treated?

Treatment depends on the cause:

- Normal newborn discharge requires no treatment and resolves on its own.
- Irritation or vulvovaginitis may be managed by improving hygiene, avoiding perfumed products, and using barrier creams, such as petroleum jelly.
- Infections may require a short course of topical or oral antibiotics or antifungals.
- If a foreign body is suspected, a specialist, such as a paediatric gynaecologist, may need to remove it.

Prevention

Here are some tips to prevent vaginal irritation and abnormal discharge:

- Teach children to wipe front to back as soon as they are able.
- Use plain water or gentle, fragrance-free cleansers during baths.
- Avoid bubble baths, harsh soaps, and heavily fragranced wipes.
- Choose cotton underwear and avoid overly tight clothes.
- Ensure nappies are changed frequently to keep the area clean and dry.

Vaginal discharge in babies and toddlers is usually a normal part of development or a response to mild irritation. Most cases do not indicate a serious problem and resolve with simple hygiene

WORMS

If you have ever encountered me on social media, you'll know I love a good parasite! Which is why it is fitting that the last thing I write about in this book is worms.

> **MY STORY**
>
> I will never forget the moment I discovered my child had worms. Somehow, I doubt she will either. She had been off form for about two weeks: not sleeping well, eating less than usual, and complaining of a sore tummy. One night, I went in to kiss her goodnight and discovered her scratching her bum. I had an 'Aha!' moment, turned on the torch of my mobile phone, and inspected the vicinity. Well, there they all were – little white worms waving up at me. I'm pretty sure my shrieks were heard in the next county, and such was my alarm that my poor daughter started wailing. It was a chaotic, memorable moment. My husband was dispatched to the local late-night pharmacy, because those visitors were *not* welcome in my home for one second longer. Within an hour, every single family member was dosed with mebendazole – a type of medicine for treating worms.

Worms, also known as threadworms or pinworms, are really very common in children. Whilst they are generally not dangerous, they are unpleasant and can make your child feel pretty rotten.

How do children catch worms?

Threadworms (also called pinworms) are caught by swallowing their eggs. These microscopic eggs can live on hands, surfaces, toys, clothing, and bedding for up to two weeks. Here's a typical scenario:

- Child 1, who has worms, scratches their itchy bottom at night.
- Eggs get onto their fingers.
- Those fingers go onto toys, door handles, or into mouths (theirs or a sibling's).
- Child 2 swallows the eggs, and the cycle starts all over again.

Schools and childcare settings are prime spots for spread, but it's nobody's fault, and it doesn't mean your home is unclean.

Symptoms

The most common sign of worms? An itchy bottom, especially at night. You might also notice:

- restless sleep
- irritability or tiredness during the day
- loss of appetite
- occasionally, tummy ache or nausea
- sometimes, you may even spot tiny white worms in the poo or around your child's bottom.

Not every child has symptoms, which is why worms spread so easily in families.

How is it treated?

The good news is that treatment is simple. The most commonly used medicine is called mebendazole. It's available without prescription for children over two years of age. For under-twos, chat to your GP for tailored advice.

Key points to remember:

- Treat everyone in the household, even if they're not itchy.
- A second dose of medicine after two weeks is often recommended, just in case eggs have hatched since the first treatment.
- Don't worry if you don't see dead worms after treatment. They pass in the poo and may not be visible.

Worms can be treated at home, but contact your GP if:

- your child is under two years old
- there's ongoing discomfort despite treatment
- you see blood in your child's stool or they complain of significant pain.

Stopping the cycle

Medication kills the worms, but it doesn't kill the eggs. That's where hygiene steps in. For the next two weeks, you'll need to go into 'worm-busting mode'.

Daily tips

- Wash hands thoroughly with soap and warm water, especially after using the toilet and before eating. Use a nail brush to clean under the nails.
- Keep nails short and clean. Try to discourage nail-biting or thumb-sucking.

- Bathe your child first thing in the morning to remove eggs laid overnight.
- Pop on snug-fitting underwear or pyjamas at night to help prevent scratching.

Around the house

- Wash bedding, towels, and pyjamas regularly – hot washes if possible.
- Clean bathroom surfaces, light switches, and door handles daily.
- Vacuum bedrooms and living areas often.
- Try not to shake out bedding or clothes, it can spread eggs into the air.

Remember, your child can have worms even if you haven't seen them. They generally only come out at night to lay their eggs. My children had enough symptoms of worms on later occasions for me to treat them without ever going looking for proof of their existence again. But if you are in the mood for grossing yourself out, yes, the best time to spot them is at nighttime.

Acknowledgements

I want to acknowledge my parents, John and Maura, who raised me with the values of kindness and compassion.

Special thanks to my immediate and wider family for putting up with several months of plans sacrificed for 'the book' and supporting me through almost a year of researching and writing.

Thank you to Professor Colin Hawkes who read through the manuscript and gave very helpful suggestions.

To my friends, especially my book club pals, the Lit Chicks, who always said I had a book in me – thanks for cheering me on.

Thank you to the team in Hachette for your amazing support. Ciara, Catherine and Joanna – you are all talented and very patient women!

And finally, to my mentor, Professor Anthony (Tony) Ryan, sadly no longer with us. Tony, you told me to write and see where it took me. Thank you, Tony.

Image credits

Book Illustrations by Aoibhe Cubie

Photo section

Page 1, top image: Shutterstock/Skylines
Page 1, bottom image: Science Photo Library
Page 2: Shutterstock/Sukjai Photo
Page 3, top image: Shutterstock/Lukassek
Page 3, bottom image: Dr. P. Marazzi/Science Photo Library
Page 4, top image: iStock/sruilk
Page 4, middle: iStock/Helin Loik-Tomson
Page 4, bottom: Science Photo Library
Page 5, top: iStock/Surasak Suwanmake
Page 5, bottom: iStock/thebaikers
Page 6, top: Shutterstock/Tanapat Lek.Jiw
Page 6, bottom: Shutterstock/Alfasatryapermana
Page 7, top: Shutterstock/cha_cha
Page 7, bottom: Rini Rezeki
Page 8, top: Shutterstock/Phichet Chaiyabin
Page 8, bottom: author's own

Resources

HSE (Health Service Executive, Ireland) www.hse.ie

Children's Health Ireland www.childrenshealthireland.ie

NHS (National Health Service, UK) www.nhs.co.uk

World Health Organisation www.who.int

Parentline Ireland, a confidential helpline for parents and guardians www.parentline.ie 01-8733500

Samaritans www.samaritans.org 116123 or email jo@samaritans.ie (Ireland)/jo@samaritans.org (UK)

Cry-sis Helpline (UK, for parents of babies who cry excessively) www.cry-sis.org.uk 080044807 37

The Lullaby Trust, a charity that exists to keep babies safe during sleep and keep grieving families supported www.lullabytrust.org.uk

UK Sling Consortium https://babyslingsafety.co.uk

Association of Lactation Consultants in Ireland www.alcireland.ie

AsIAm, Ireland's national autism charity www.asiam.ie

Irish Society for Autism www.autism.ie

Inclusion Ireland, which advocates for people with intellectual disabilities www.inclusionireland.ie

Rare Ireland, a charity for children with rare genetic conditions www.rareireland.ie

ERIC: The Children's Bowel & Bladder Charity (UK) www.eric.org.uk

National Poisons Information Centre (Ireland) www.poisons.ie and 01-809 2166

The Children and Young People's Cancer Association (CCLG, UK) www.cclg.org.uk

DermNet, a free dermatology resource with information on skin conditions and rashes www.dermnetnz.org

STARS, a charity with resources on anoxic seizures www.heartrhythmalliance.org/stars

First aid training courses available from:
Red Cross Ireland www.redcross.ie
Red Cross UK www.redcross.org.uk
St John Ambulance (Ireland) www.stjohn.ie
Order of Malta (Ireland) www.orderofmaltaireland.org

Index

1-2 years 130-153
accidents 144-153
common cold 150-151
developmental milestones 136-139
falls 144-150
faltering growth 136
feeding 130-135
growth 135-136
illnesses 144-153
red flags 148, 152-153
sleep 139-141
vaccines 141-144
2-5 years 154-193
accidents 2-5, 179-191
developmental milestones 164-168
ear infections 180-182
feeding 154-157
growth 157-163
illnesses 179-191
red flags 167, 182, 184
sleep 174-179
tantrums 171-174
2-6 weeks 40-65
colic 57-59
crying 57-59

developmental milestones 51-53
feeding 40-45
illnesses 49, 63
pee 48-49
red flags 45-46, 58, 63-65
sleep 53-55
4-6 months 100-101
developmental milestones 91-93
eczema 89-90
feeding 82-86
illnesses 95-103
pee 86-87
poop 86-87
skin 87-91
sleep 93-94
sleep safety 94
vaccines 95
6-12 months 104-129
accidents 117-129
choking 118-123
developmental milestones 110-114
feeding 104-108
growth 108-109
illnesses 117-129

386 | SHOULD I BE WORRIED?

A
accidents
  1–2 years 144–153
  2–5 years 2–5, 179–191
  6–12 months 117–129
ADD/ADHD 212–213
adenoids 294–297
adenovirus 100
ages
  0–5 11–12
  1–2 years 130–153
  2–5 years 154–193
  2–6 weeks 40–65
  4–6 months 100–101
  6–12 months 104–129
  7–12 weeks 66–81
  first 24 hours 13–19
  first week 19–39
allergies 297–302
autism 213–215

B
baby carriers 55–57
babyproofing 117–118, 128–129
baby teeth 276–278
bacterial illnesses
  4–6 months 101–103
  bedwetting 178–179, 302–305
Benign Neonatal Sleep Myoclonus 247–249
birthmarks 33–34
brain tumours 238–241
breath-holding 249–250
breathing
  first 24 hours 14–15
  problems 305–307
Brief Resolved Unexplained Events 78–79
bronchiolitis 152

C
car seats 38–39
chest infections 152
chickenpox 287–288, 307–310
choking 310–315
6–12 months 118–123
circumcision 189–191
cold sores 287
colic 317–321
common cold
  1–2 years 150–151
  2–6 weeks 57–59
constipation 198, 204–206
contact dermatitis 292
cow's milk 130–132
CPR 315–317
cradle cap 91
croup 152, 322–324
crying
  2–6 weeks 57–59
  first 24 hours 17
  first week 26
cystic fibrosis 35

pee 109–110
poo 109–110
skin 117
sleep 114–116
7–12 weeks 66–81
developmental milestones 70–72
faltering growth 67–69
feeding 66–69
illnesses 77
pee 70
poo 69–71
red flags 79–80
sleep 72
vaccines 72–76

INDEX | 387

D

developmental delays 324–327
developmental differences 209–220
developmental milestones
1–2 years 136–139
2–5 years 164–168
2–6 weeks 51–53
4–6 months 91–93
6–12 months 110–114
7–12 weeks 70–72
diarrhoea 200
doctors' appointments 267–274
dyspraxia 211–212

E

ear infections 151
2–5 years 180–182
eczema 283–285, 292, 327–330
4–6 months 89–90
epilepsy 226–232
eye issues 330–333

F

fainting 247–266
falls 144–150
faltering growth 42–43
1–2 years 136
7–12 weeks 67–69
febrile convulsions, see febrile seizures
feeding 280
1–2 years 130–135
2–5 years 154–157
2–6 weeks 40–45
4–6 months 82–86
6–12 months 104–108
7–12 weeks 66–69
first 24 hours 15–16

G

gastroenteritis 337–339
genitalia 50–51, see also unde-scended testicles
grommets 181–182

functional abdominal pain 200–201
4–6 months 83
2–5 years 154–155
food allergies
follow-on formula 105
fits 247–266
sleep 25–26
skin 27
red flags 23, 24, 26, 31
rashes 27
poop 24
pee 25
head shape 31–33
feeding 20–23
crying 26
first week 19–39
CPR 315–317
first-aid courses 118
falls 123
choking 118–119, 311–315
burns 126–127
first aid
sleep 17
skin 18
poop 16
pee 16–17
health checks 18, 35–38
feeding 15–16
crying 17
breathing 14–15
first 24 hours 13–19
fever 334–337
weaning 106–108
first week 20–23

growth
1-2 years 135-136
2-5 years 157-163
6-12 months 108-109

H
hair issues 339-343
hand, foot, and mouth disease 286
hayfever 343-345
head lice 345-348
head shape
7-12 weeks 76-77
first week 31-33
health checks 18, see also screening tests
herpes simplex virus 287
hip dysplasia 37-38
hospital visits 267-274

I
illnesses
1-2 years 144-153
2-5 years 179-191
2-6 weeks 63
4-6 months 95-103
6-12 months 117-129
7-12 weeks 77
impetigo 288
infant shuddering spells 258-261

J
jaundice 27

L
language 166-167
leukaemia 232-235
lymphoma 235-238
Lynch, Dr Niamh 1-9

M
measles 288, 348-351
meltdowns 171-174
meningitis 285
molluscum contagiosum 289

N
nappy rash 351-354
napping 175
4-6 months 88-89
neuroblastoma 243-246
neurodivergence 209-210
diagnosis 216-218
early signs 215-218
supporting your child 219

O
overeating 199

P
pee
2-6 weeks 48-49
4-6months 86-87
6-12 months 109-110
7-12 weeks 70
first 24 hours 16-17
first week 25
personal stories
ADD/ADHD 212
autism 213-215
brain tumours 238-241
breath-holding spells 250
colic 60-62
dyspraxia 211
epilepsy 226-227
falls 148-150
febrile seizures 254-255
hospital visits 267-269
infant shuddering spells 258
leukaemia 232

INDEX | 389

lymphoma 235-238
neuroblastoma 243
reflex anoxic seizures 251
sensory processing disorder 210
tics 261
Wilms tumour 241
worms 376
picky eating 133-135
poisoning 355-356
poop, *see also* toilet training
4-6 months 86-87
6-12 months 109-110
7-12 weeks 69-71
first 24 hours 16
first week 24
projectile vomiting 23
psoriasis 292
PURPLE crying 318

R

rashes 283-293
first week 27
infectious 285-291
nappy rash 88-89, 351-354
non-infectious 291-293
red flags 102, 145
1-2 years 148, 152-153
2-5 years 167, 182, 184
2-6 weeks 45-46, 58, 63-65
4-6 months 85, 96-97
6-12 months 119, 124-126
7-12 weeks 79-80
breathing problems 306
chickenpox 309
colic 320
croup 324
eczema 330
eye issues 333
febrile seizures 256
fever 335-336

S

scabies 289-291
scarlet fever 286-287
screening tests 35-38, *see also* health checks
seizures 226-232
febrile seizures 254-258
reflex anoxic seizures 251-254
sensory processing disorder 210-211
sepsis 357-359
serious concerns 221-246
skin 283-293
4-6 months 87-91
6-12 months 117
first 24 hours 18
first week 27
slapped cheek syndrome 285-286
sleep
1-2 years 139-141
2-5 years 174-179
2-6 weeks 53-55
4-6 months 93-94
6-12 months 114-116

T
tantrums 171-174
teething 275-282
teething troubles 151
temperature, checking 29-30
thrush 351-354
tics 261-265
toilet training 169-171, 206,
  see also pood
tongue-tie 20-22
tonsillitis 183-185, 363-365
tooth decay 280-281
trapped wind 198
tummy troubles 197-208
  and emotions 201
  causes 198-203
  tummy upset 151
  type 1 diabetes 222-226

U
umbilical cord 18, 28-29
undescended testicles 366-368,
  see also genitalia
urinary tract infections 187-189
  2-6 weeks 49
  4-6 months 103
urticaria 291-292

V
vaccine hesitancy 74-76, 143-144
vaccines 191-192, 368-372
  1-2 years 141-144
  4-6 months 95
  7-12 weeks 72-76
  chickenpox 310
  MMR 350
  schedule 368-370
  vaginal discharge 373-376
  viral illnesses 96-101
  viral infections 199
Vitamin D 23-24
Vitamin K 19

W
weaning 106-108
  what to expect
  ages 0-5 11-12
wheezing 185-187
Wilms tumour 241-243
worms 376-379

7-12 weeks 72
first 24 hours 17
first week 25-26
sleep safety 94
sudden infant death syndrome
  360-363
supplements 160-163